Problems in
Geriatric Medicine

Problems in Practice Series

Problems in Practice Series

Series Editors : J.Fry K.Williams M.Lancaster-Smith

Problems in Geriatric Medicine

Anthony Martin
MD

Consultant Physician
Department of Geriatric Medicine
Crawley Hospital, Sussex

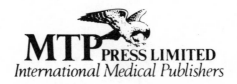

MTP PRESS LIMITED
International Medical Publishers

Published by
MTP Press Limited
Falcon House
Lancaster, England

Copyright © 1981 A. Martin

First published 1981

ISBN 0-85200-319-6

Phototypesetting by Swiftpages Limited, Liverpool and printed
by Redwood Burn Limited, Trowbridge

Contents

Preface

The fact that there are special problems in the care of the elderly in the community is ample justification for writing a separate volume on the subject. The knowledge that there are increasing numbers of older people in virtually every country in the world makes it all the more important that the family physician should have sympathy with and understanding of the problems of them, since they are likely to make up a significant part of his workload and, increasingly, will take up more of his time and energy.

There is a progressive amount of disability with advancing years, and this is particularly true of those aged 75 years and over. Increasing age is associated with serious impairment of hearing and vision, senses which younger people take for granted. Old age sees the arrival of major diseases of middle age with much greater frequency, such as ischaemic heart and cerebrovascular disease, diabetes mellitus and osteoarthritis. There are other disorders that are virtually confined to the elderly, such as fractures of the femoral neck, Paget's disease and myeloma. We now know that the disintegration of the conducting tissue of the heart is largely an age-related phenomenon. Ageing processes affect every major organ system in the body and the impairment of physiological performance resulting from these affects the elderly individual's response to infections, disease and environmental changes in complex ways that are not seen in younger people.

It is important to remember that it is not always that the disease is measurable, but the effect that the disease has on the lifestyle of the individual that really matters. These factors not only add greatly to the clinical interest of the physician, but require of him special skills in the management of the elderly patient. This book is designed to evaluate some of the problems peculiar to older patients and to assist the family physician in the management of these in the home environment. It does not pretend to be a comprehensive text book of geriatric medicine; many disorders are discussed only briefly and others omitted, not because they are necessarily unimportant, but because they have little relevance to the problems encountered in everyday family practice. Management of the older patient is essentially a practical matter and this book approaches the subject from a problem-orientated point of view.

Acknowledgements

It is only when this section is written that one realizes how much one is dependent on others. A great number of people have helped me during the relatively short gestation period of this book, and it is impossible to mention all by name.

Dr Martin Reay-Jones and Dr John Merritt have very kindly read through the draft chapters as they have poured off my typewriter and have given me the great benefit of their many years in family practice. Dr John Fry has, as always, been most helpful in making sure that I have kept strictly to the realms of my subject and not wandered into the unnecessary minutiae of geriatric medicine.

Dr Roger Briggs, now Senior Lecturer in Geriatric Medicine at Southampton University, very kindly contributed the majority of the chapter on incontinence. His expertise is so much greater than mine in this field that it would have been a pity to have omitted his contribution in a book that is, otherwise, all my own responsibility.

For some years now we have been running a vocational training scheme in Crawley for doctors going into family practice. I have learnt a lot both from my other trainer colleagues and from those young doctors who have participated in the scheme. Indeed, this book is based on our mutual experience in running a busy acute medical unit for the elderly.

Barbara Green and Una Allman have been a great help to me on the secretarial side and I am much indebted to them.

Finally I must thank my wife, who has not only corrected my grammar and read through both drafts and proofs, but has cheerfully accepted my absences during the preparation of this book.

Series Foreword

This series of books is designed to help general practitioners. So are other books. What is unusual in this instance is their collective authorship; they are written by specialists working at district general hospitals. The writers derive their own experience from a range of cases less highly selected than those on which textbooks are traditionally based. They are also in a good position to pick out topics which they see creating difficulties for the practitioners of their district, whose personal capacities are familiar to them; and to concentrate on contexts where mistakes are most likely to occur. They are all well-accustomed to working in consultation.

All the authors write from hospital experience and from the viewpoint of their specialty. There are, therefore, matters important to family practice which should be sought not within this series, but elsewhere. Within the series much practical and useful advice is to be found with which the general practitioner can compare his existing performance and build in new ideas and improved techniques.

These books are attractively produced and I recommend them.

J. P. Horder OBE
President, The Royal College
of General Practitioners

1 Demographic and social factors

Population profiles of the elderly in Great Britain – Population profiles in the United States of America – The ageing population in Eastern countries – Some considerations of the ageing process – Some special features of disease in the elderly – Myocardial infarction

The increase in the proportion of people aged over 65 years in the community is not only a phenomenon of Western society but is to be found in Eastern countries as well. What is, perhaps, more significant from the point of view of health care, is that the number of people of over 75 years is rising even more greatly in proportion to the total population. The reasons for these facts in civilized societies are not difficult to understand. In the last 70 years there has been a reduction in the death rates in all age groups under 65 years, most marked in the first year of life. For example, in Great Britain at the time of the 1851 census the death rate in children aged 0–1 year was 153 per thousand live births. The impact of public health measures, such as the Sewage and Sanitation Act and the Smallpox Vaccination Act, at the end of the last century started to reduce the childhood mortality and by 1941 there had been a reduction in the death rate of children 0–1 years to 58 per thousand live births. The current death rate for the same age group is now below 18 per thousand live births. This has meant that a male infant born now is expected to live to the age of 68.8 years and a female to 74.8 years.

Reduced
death rate

Dramatic declines in death rates in the elderly have not been achieved in the same period of time. A man aged 65 years at the time of the 1851 census had an expectation of life of ten years and in the following 120 years this had only increased by two years despite all the advances in medical and public health techniques.

Population profiles of the elderly in Great Britain

Reduced birth rate

At the present time there are almost 8 million people over the age of 65 years, who represent about 14% of the total population. There are about 3 million people over the age of 75 years. Three fifths of the elderly are women. Projections suggest that the elderly population will continue to increase in Great Britain for the next ten years and then fall off slightly. Because of the falling birth rate of the last few years the percentage of the elderly population will increase and is likely to be about 20% by the end of the century.

Table 1.1   The changing elderly population in Great Britain

| Year | Total numbers (millions) | | | |
	65–74	75–84	85 and over	Total over 65
1970	4.5	2.0	0.3	6.8
1980	4.8	2.4	0.6	7.8
1990	4.7	2.7	0.8	8.2
2000	4.5	2.7	0.9	8.1

(Projected. O.P.C.S.)

The medical problems that one can expect from this large elderly age group are, of course, difficult to quantify. However, it has been estimated that 13% of those aged 65 years and over are physically handicapped in the sense that their living activities are severely restricted. Just over 4% of the elderly people living at home are permanently bed-fast or housebound. In the '85-year-old and over' age group this figure rises to 20%. When one adds to these figures the incidence of mental illness, namely 10% of the over 65s being demented, one half of these severely, it is clear that the medical problems that are likely to involve the family physician are very great indeed.

Population profiles in the United States of America

Here one sees a very similar picture to that in Great Britain, although the proportion of people over 65 years is slightly lower.

Table 1.2 Population projections, USA 1975–2050

Year	Total numbers (millions) *with % of whole population in brackets*		
	65–74	75 and over	Total over 65 years
1975	13.9 (6.5%)	8.4 (3.9%)	22.3 (10.4%)
1990	17.5 (7.1%)	11.4 (4.7%)	8.9 (11.8%)
2000	17.1 (6.5%)	13.5 (5.1%)	30.6 (11.7%)
2050	29.1 (9.2%)	22.1 (6.9%)	51.2 (16.1%)

Ideally the objective of care of the elderly is to preserve for individuals as much freedom of choice as possible in the way they wish to spend their life. However, social changes in Western society have narrowed this choice to some degree. The availability of work for the elderly has diminished in times of increasing general unemployment. Modern industrial society has led to a drift in the responsibility for the elderly away from the family. They can no longer count, as a matter of right and of moral and legal obligation, on economic support from their children. The elderly now come to rely on voluntary and State organizations for help rather than on the family. A survey in England in 1976 showed that 28% of the elderly lived alone at home and a further 41% lived with only the spouse. Only 12% of those over 65 years lived with their children. Figures from the US Bureau of the Census, 1976, suggest that a very similar situation exists in the United States. All these factors make the work of family physicians that much more difficult and have, perhaps, tended to push older people towards home and hospital accommodation, situations in which the old person will lose much of his remaining independence. For purely economic reasons, let alone moral ones, it is unlikely that any society will be able to stand continued pressure for increasing residential accommodation. The family physician has an important part to play in the redevelopment of a society in which the elderly can remain safely and independently at home.

Marginal note: Unemployment

Marginal note: Diminished family support

The ageing population in Eastern countries

The situation in Eastern countries is rather different to that in Europe and the United States. Although the numbers of elderly people are growing rapidly, partly as a result of improved health care, the birth rate in most of these countries continues to be very high despite vigorous efforts on the part of Governments to reduce them. As a result the proportion of elderly people in the total population remains at about 5%.

13

Japan

Low birth rate

However, in Japan a very different state of affairs exists since there has been a precipitous drop in the birth rate since 1950, so that now Japan has the second lowest birth rate in the world. This fact combined with greatly improved standards of health care and the increased life-expectancy of old people has led to the beginnings of a very steep rise in the proportion of elderly people. The present percentage of those aged 65 years and over in Japan is now about 8% and this will more than double by the beginning of the next century. In fact, the elderly population explosion in Japan is likely to be more rapid than in any country in history.

Loss of family support

Rural elderly

Early retirement

There are three important factors that will be of great concern to the Japanese health services. It is likely that the great tradition of family care for the aged will break down partially, if not totally, which will add further stress to medical and social services. The ageing population live largely in rural areas, but there has been a massive flight of younger people from the rural areas to the cities in the past few years and this will put great geographical strains on services. Finally, it has been the custom in Japan to retire people early in large industrial enterprises, and although it is known that a large proportion of Japanese would like to continue to work into old age, it is unlikely that they will be able to do so unless they take up self-employment.

Thus the problems of an increased proportion of elderly people in the community are not confined to westernized societies. It is likely that by the end of the century there will be an almost universal increase in the number of elderly to be supported by a diminishing proportion of people of working age. Some of the dimensions of these problems can already be seen in some societies; these will increase and extend to others.

Some considerations of the ageing process

Genetic factors

Although it has been the subject of considerable research, the mechanism of ageing in the body is still poorly understood. There is no single satisfactory model that explains ageing processes throughout the body. Genetic factors are clearly important in the ageing process and as in so many other aspects of life, it is important to choose one's parents carefully! There are some theories based on the deterioration of protein synthesizing mechanisms, for example, abnormalities of DNA and RNA. Certainly we know that toxic chemicals and radiation may

14

damage protein synthesis and cause mutations, and increasing mutations may shorten the longevity of animals, but there appears to be a fundamental difference between the mutations normally attributable to ageing and those caused by external factors.

Hayflick phenomenon

A few years ago Hayflick showed that fibroblasts grown in tissue culture had a set number of divisions before they died, a sort of biological clock. However, other workers have been unable to simulate these findings in less artificial circumstances and this theory has now to some extent fallen into disrepute.

Auto-immune theory

There appears to be increasing immunological incompetence as age advances. The cells responsible for defence and repair, the lymphocytes and fibroblasts, may undergo mutation and result in antigenically altered cell proteins. This may in turn lead to two changes, (1) the possibility of an immune response being set up against them and (2) mutation within lymphocytes themselves can give rise to clones of lymphocytic cells with potential auto-immune pathogenicity. There is a decline in the T-cells with age and this is associated with a rise in the incidence of infections and malignancies. The B-lymphocytes which develop into plasma cells increase with age and there is a progressive rise in the plasma immunoglobulins, which explains the rise of the ESR with age and the much higher incidence of myeloma and giant cell arteritis in the elderly.

Cellular fall out

It has long been thought that one of the causes of ageing is the progressive loss of cells throughout the body, but this fact may be erroneous because of sampling error and there may not be steady cell death.

Hormones

Although hormonal influences do control some of the changes associated with age, for example, senile osteoporosis as a result of diminished oestrogen secretion, there is no direct proof that dysfunction of one or more endocrine glands leads to whole body ageing.

External factors

There are small isolated communities throughout the world in which some people live to very advanced ages. This is seen in the Ecuadorian Andes, and some remote areas of the USSR and the Pakistan/China borders. There is a very low population density in all these places. Also the people take a diet low in animal fats, have a high degree of physical activity and also have the possible genetic advantage of longevity. When these people move to other areas they appear to lose much of their potential longevity, whether as a result of dietary changes or exposure to new infections, or other factors.

Some special features of disease in the elderly

Most of the special features of disease in the elderly are a result of the structural and functional changes that occur with ageing.

The effects of ageing

Nephron loss

Hepatic function

Neurone loss

Atheroma

Heart conducting tissue

Amyloid

The maintenance and repair of body tissues becomes progressively less efficient as age advances. Diminution of physiological performance can be demonstrated in most organ systems. There is continual loss of nephrons in the kidney with resultant deficiency in renal function. This may not be easily demonstrable by ordinary renal function tests, but there is significant loss of ability to excrete many drugs, such as digoxin, which may account for the increased sensitivity to these drugs in the elderly. Hepatic function also declines and this, too, has some relevance to drug treatment in older patients. There is neurone loss in the brain, degenerative changes in the autonomic nervous system and reduction in nerve conduction velocity with increasing age. Changes in the lungs account for the diminished maximum oxygen uptake that is clearly demonstrable in the elderly. Cellular loss in the pancreas may account for the great increase in the incidence of diabetes mellitus. The acceleration of atheromatous changes with age results in the increased prevalence of strokes and ischaemic heart disease, as well as the appearance of vascular phenomena that do not occur in younger people, such as mesenteric artery ischaemia. Cellular loss in the conducting tissue of the heart produces an increasingly high incidence of sino-atrial and atrio-ventricular node dysfunction, features that are rarely seen below the age of 70 years. Deposits of amyloid in the heart are specifically a problem of senescence.

Impairment of homeostasis

Hypothermia
Postural hypotension

With increasing age there is less ability to react to stress and changes in the external environment. Temperature regulation becomes impaired and hypothermia becomes a real problem for the older patient. Postural hypotension is seen much more frequently in the elderly as a result of either degenerative changes in the autonomic nervous system or of the increased sensitivity to many drugs.

Altered reaction to drugs

Problems with drug sensitivity are extremely common in old age. This is probably largely due to impairment of drug

16

metabolism and excretion, but may also be a result of increased sensitivity of the target organ.

Altered reaction to infection and stress

Transient, but often severe, mental confusion presents many problems in the elderly. This is usually a result of stress or infection, but may be initiated by any generalized illness or even environmental changes. Major disease, such as cardiac infarction, may be painless and present purely as a confusional state.

Multiple pathological processes

One is rarely dealing with a single disease process in the elderly and indeed, it has been said that if one diagnoses only a single disease in the elderly at least one other is being missed! This is a result of the coincidence of so many degenerative diseases and to the accumulation of illness.

Unrecognized problems

Many surveys of elderly populations have shown that there is much disease and disability that is not reported to the family physician. Disturbances of locomotor function, anaemia, depression and dementia, as well as failing vision and hearing, may only come to light when the patient suffers some major accident or sudden illness, such as a stroke. By constant surveillance of his elderly patients the family physician is in a good position to alleviate many of these problems, although routine screening procedures in the elderly are probably not economically viable or morally desirable.

Management

The family physician needs to be able to differentiate between the acceptable disability of ageing and the unacceptable disabilities of illness in the elderly. The grey area between these two is often very difficult to identify, but this critical area is one in which the family physician is in a unique position to assess and, if necessary, modify.

The other factors in management that are particularly important in the elderly concern the multiplicity of disease and disability that occur and are inextricably linked in older people. The family physician will be able to recognize the medical and social factors that concern the independence of his elderly

patients better than anybody else and, with a sound understanding of these, and an optimistic and sympathetic attitude,
should be able to influence favourably their quality of life.

Disorders of the cardiovascular system (I)

MYOCARDIAL AND VALVULAR DISEASE; BLOOD PRESSURE

Pathophysiology of the myocardium – Measured high blood pressure – The differential diagnosis of myocardial infarction – Valvular heart disease – Heart failure – The differential diagnosis of swollen legs

Heart disease in the elderly is one of the commonest problems that will be encountered in general practice. The mortality rate from heart disease rises with age and accounts for more than a third of deaths over the age of 65 years in the Western world. The morbidity rate from heart disease in the elderly is imposs-ible to quantify, but as the incidence of cardiac abnormalities in the 65–74 year age group may be as high as 50% and in the over 75-year-olds around 60%, it is likely that a significant number of these people will suffer some limitation of their activities or at least symptoms of dyspnoea, angina or oedema of the legs. The major diseases of ageing in the heart are myocardial in-farction, angina, rhythm and conduction abnormalities and to a lesser extent valvular disease. Heart disease in itself is not only likely to contribute to morbidity in the elderly but is also a significant factor in limiting the rehabilitation of patients with other problems, such as after strokes and fractured femurs.

Pathophysiology of the myocardium

Brown atrophy The classical description of brown atrophy of the myocardium may well represent a normal ageing process. In this situation there is wasting of the heart muscle with a decrease of heart

19

weight and histologically there is an accumulation of lipofuscin in the myocardial cells. There is, however, very little evidence that brown atrophy gives rise to myocardial dysfunction.

Fibrosis
Fibrosis of the myocardium has been shown to be of two types. Large lesions, greater than 2 cm long, are found in association with coronary artery disease. They are more common in men than women and probably represent small myocardial infarcts. The small lesions, less than 2 cm in length, are probably the result of focal myocarditis caused by healing areas of infection. These small lesions are common in the elderly and may affect the conducting tissue of the heart.

Senile cardiac amyloidosis
Senile cardiac amyloidosis appears to be an age-related disease and can be found in 12% of men over the age of 80 years. The amyloid deposits may be in the atrium or the ventricle but are not usually associated with deposits elsewhere in the body. Senile cardiac amyloidosis may cause both cardiac arrhythmias and heart failure, but it can really only be accurately diagnosed at autopsy. It is included here both for completeness and to illustrate the complexity of myocardial pathology in the elderly.

Others
Other cardiomyopathies in the elderly are rare, but primary myocardial disease may occur as a result of thiamine (vitamin B_1) deficiency and this is probably also the cause of alcoholic cardiomyopathy.

Myocardial infarction

Ischaemic heart disease is the single most important form of heart disease in the elderly and in one population study was found to present in 12% of women and 20% of men over the age of 65 years. As age increases the preponderance of men with this condition gradually disappears and indeed, the mortality rate for this condition is equal for the two sexes at the age of 80 years.

Chest pain
The presenting symptom of myocardial infarction in the elderly is usually, but by no means always, retrosternal chest pain. This may be variously described as 'crushing', 'constricting', 'aching' or 'like a heavy weight'. The pain is usually demonstrated by the patient by passing his hand horizontally across the lower chest, but sometimes it may be across the upper abdomen or even the upper part of the thorax. More rarely the only site of pain may be in the neck or lower jaws and may mimic toothache. The pain may radiate to the back, the shoulders or down the arms. There is some evidence that

20

myocardial infarction may present without pain and the incidence of this increases with advancing age. The sudden onset

Dyspnoea

of dyspnoea is an important symptom of myocardial infarction and this may occur at any time, but paroxysmal nocturnal dyspnoea is especially common and one should always exclude a silent myocardial infarction in this situation. Occasionally myocardial infarction may present as a stroke. Sometimes the

Syncope
asymptomatic

only symptom of myocardial infarction is a syncopal episode or merely the onset of severe dizziness and weakness. In a few patients there may be no symptoms at all and the diagnosis is only detected when a routine electrocardiogram is performed. As always with the elderly, history-taking may be considerably modified by short-term memory loss and confusion, and it is essential to interview relatives and friends as well as the patient. There is no doubt that these factors make the diagnosis of heart disease more difficult in older people and probably accounts largely for the reported high incidence of silent infarction in old age.

Diagnosis

The diagnosis of myocardial infarction should be made confidently on the history in most cases, but there are certain cardinal features on clinical examination, the electrocardiogram (e.c.g.) and blood investigation that will confirm the diagnosis. Clinical examination may reveal a patient with signs

Shock
Fever

of shock and dyspnoea at rest. The temperature is usually raised. There may be abnormalities of the pulse, both in its volume and rhythm. There may be hypotension, but in some patients the blood pressure may actually be raised. The cardiac

Rhythm
abnormalities

rhythm may be slow if there is involvement of the conduction tissue and there is a degree of heart block or sinus bradycardia. Irregularities of the heart are common and are usually due to ventricular or supraventricular ectopic beats, but atrial fibrillation may often be a direct result of infarction. Auscultation of the heart often helps to elucidate the rhythm abnormalities and there may be a fourth heart sound, indicating a degree of left ventricular failure. More rarely a pericardial rub may be heard. Sometimes left ventricular infarction may result in damage to the papillary muscle and lead to free mitral valvular regurgitation, in which case a loud, mid-systolic murmur with an ejection click is heard at the apex and may be radiated widely over the praecordium. Other signs of left ventricular failure are the presence of an elevated jugular venous pressure and finding of crepitations at the lung bases.

Electrocardio-
gram

The 12 lead e.c.g. is an essential investigation in anyone who may be suspected of having a myocardial infarction. The

21

classic changes of an infarction on the e.c.g. should be well-known: a full-thickness infarct produces a Q wave, which is defined as the first negative deflection wider than 0.04 s (or one small square on standard e.c.g. paper), an elevated S–T segment and a biphasic and 'later' inverted T wave.

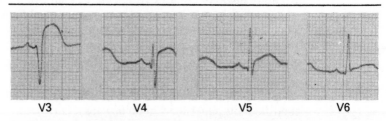

V3   V4   V5   V6

Acute antero-septal myocardial infarction

Figure 2.1

These changes are usually seen immediately but may in some instances be delayed for several hours. As the infarction process progresses the raised S–T take-off falls towards the iso-electric line and the T wave becomes symmetrically inverted. A partial thickness or subendocardial infarct will not produce Q waves, and the signs here are of sharp symmetrical T wave inversion.

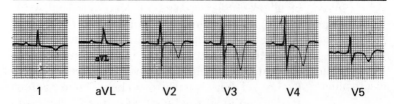

1   aVL   V2   V3   V4   V5

Acute antero-septal subendocardial infarction

Figure 2.2

In rare instances none of these e.c.g. changes are seen, but there are usually other changes which will suggest the diagnosis. A left bundle branch block pattern may be seen and here the QRS complexes are widened to 0.12 s or greater and there is left axis deviation. This finding is especially useful if the abnormality was not seen prior to the infarction. Since Rosenbaum described the trifascicular nature of the conducting system of the heart a few years ago, it has become appreciated that lesser degrees of heart block may indicate infarction, and in particular the appearance of left anterior hemiblock may be the only e.c.g. sign of myocardial infarction, and indeed is an important factor in considering the manage-

Blood tests

ment of the patient. Heart block is discussed in more detail in Chapter 3.

Blood investigations have a very useful place in both the diagnostic and, to a lesser extent, the prognostic assessment of myocardial infarction. The peripheral blood count shows that the white cell count is raised after 24 hours and the erythrocyte sedimentation rate after about 48 hours. The cardiac enzymes are also raised, the serum glutamatic–oxolo-acetic transaminase (SGOT) starts rising after 24 hours and usually falls to normal after 4 or 5 days, the lactate dehydro-genase (LDH) tends to rise after 3 or 4 days and may remain elevated for a week or so. All these parameters bear some relation to the degree of muscle damage and to some extent give an estimate of the size of the infarct.

Table 2.1 Blood tests in myocardial infarction

Test	Days after infarction				
	1	2	3	4	5
WBC	+ +	+	+	+	
ESR		+	+ +	+ +	+
SGOT		+	+ +	+ +	+
LDH			+	+	+ +

The differential diagnosis of myocardial infarction

Reflux oesophagitis

Burning pain

This a common problem in the elderly, especially in those who are overweight. The difficulties of differential diagnosis are compounded by the frequent co-existence of this disease with ischaemic heart disease. Sometimes it is almost impossible to differentiate the pain of reflux oesophagitis with that of myocardial infarction, but usually the pain of reflux oesophagi-tis is described as 'burning' and the patient will demonstrate the distribution of the pain with a vertical sweep of his hand up and down the sternum. Digestive system pain may be local-ized around the position of the cardiac apex and, for practical purposes, any pain below the left nipple may be regarded as non-cardiac. Belching is a common symptom of cardiac, diges-tive or gallbladder disease and is of little help in differential diagnosis, except that it will rarely relieve cardiac pain. In difficult cases it is worth trying the effect of antacids and sub-lingual trinitrin respectively to see which may relieve the symptoms. A chest X-ray may show a gas bubble behind the heart, indicating a hiatus hernia, and a barium swallow X-ray may be helpful.

Dissecting aortic aneurism

Degenerative changes in the aorta may result in splitting of the wall forming a dissecting aneurysm. This frequently starts at the aortic root and may well obstruct one or more of the coronary artery ostia, and this will mimic the clinical and electrocardiographic features of myocardial infarction. Aortic dissection is frequently fatal, but on some occasions there may be dissection back into the aortic lumen without great interference with the patient's health. Aortic dissection may also involve the great arteries in the neck and cause hemiplegia. Aortic valvular incompetence will result if the valve ring is involved in the dissection.

Dissection of the aorta appears to be more frequent in patients with hypertension but is not necessarily associated with this. The clinical features are often very difficult to distinguish from acute myocardial infarction for the reasons outlined above, but the symptom of back pain should alert one to the diagnosis of dissection. There may be unequal radial pulses and the femoral pulses may be absent. The e.c.g. may be of little use if it shows evidence of acute myocardial infarction, but if it does not, then aortic dissection must be considered in the differential diagnosis of acute central chest pain. The chest X-ray is often of little help, but it may be possible to see dilatation of the aorta, and the finding of a double shadow of the aortic outline is diagnostic. Treatment is usually medical and there are very few cases that are suitable for surgical repair.

Unequal
pulses

Other diseases mimicking myocardial infarction

Pericarditis

Acute pericarditis may produce symptoms indistinguishable from myocardial infarction and is most commonly a result of a viral infection; but it may be caused by other diseases, such as neoplastic invasion of the pericardium from bronchial carcinomas, uraemia or, very rarely in the Western world, from rheumatic fever. There is usually a history of an upper respiratory tract infection with viral pericarditis and the pain frequently radiates to the shoulder. Clinically there is almost always a pericardial rub heard, although this may be quite transient and it is important to listen to the heart frequently. The e.c.g. is diagnostic and there is a high S–T take-off with a saddle shaped depression in the elevated S–T segment. There are no pathological Q waves and the changes are usually widespread and are not localized to one area of the myocardium as they are in infarction. It must be remembered, however, that acute myocardial infarction frequently shows a pericardial reaction on the e.c.g. if it is full thickness.

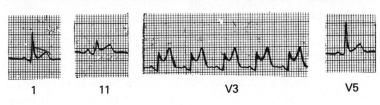

1   11   V3   V5

Acute viral pericarditis

Figure 2.3

Cholecystitis   Acute cholecystitis may occasionally be confused with myocardial infarction, but the usual finding of jaundice and right hypochondrial tenderness with the former should present few Herpes zoster   difficulties for the physician. Herpes zoster affecting one of the middle thoracic sensory roots may rarely raise suspicions of cardiac problems, but the inevitable appearance of the rash after 2 or 3 days of premonitory pain will always dispel the mystery.

The management of myocardial infarction

Control of pain   The most important immediate action to take is to control the presenting symptoms of the infarction, whether this be pain or dyspnoea. Adequate analgesia is essential and there is some evidence that rapid pain relief may limit the area of muscle damage. Diamorphine (heroin) in a dose of up to 10 mg intramuscularly should be given and this drug is preferable to either morphine or pethidine as it is less likely to cause nausea and vomiting which will make the patient even less comfortable. Whichever opiate is used, it is wise to combine it with an anti-emetic agent such as perphenazine (Fentazin) 5 mg intramuscularly or cyclizine (Valoid) 50 mg i.m., if there are signs Heart failure   of nausea. Heart failure and acute dyspnoea also require the use of adequate analgesia and the concurrent administration of intravenous frusemide (Lasix) 40–80 mg and aminophylline 0.25–0.5 g. If available the inhalation of oxygen is useful and it is worth remembering the use of 'cuffing' the legs to effect a medical venesection if there is no rapid relief of the dyspnoea. Arrhythmia   An arrhythmia may be present and exacerbate the heart failure. It is vital to identify the exact disorder with an e.c.g. before the appropriate treatment is instituted (this is discussed in Chapter 3). The use of digoxin after myocardial infarction is best avoided unless there is rapid uncontrolled atrial fibrillation.

Home or hospital

The doctor must then decide whether to admit the patient to hospital or whether to continue his treatment at home. There is little doubt that if the home circumstances are favourable and if the infarction is uncomplicated, elderly patients are best treated in their homes. The family physician is in a good position to judge this as he will usually know the family background well. If he has no e.c.g. machine or is uncertain about interpreting the tracing that he has taken, it is wise to call out the local hospital specialist to advise in the patient's home. The two doctors may then continue to manage the patient at home in consultation; this will probably entail a further visit from the hospital specialist after a week or ten days. If, however, there are any complications, such as a cardiac arrhythmia or continued pain of heart failure, it is wiser to admit the patient to hospital.

The majority of patients with myocardial infarction can be perfectly well managed at home, judged on the guidelines mentioned in the previous paragraph. These patients do not require bed rest after the first 24 hours, and early mobilization is important. For the first two or three days it is satisfactory for the patient to sit out and be free to take a few steps to a convenient lavatory or bedside commode. In this way constipation is avoided and the incidence of venous thrombosis and pulmonary embolism is minimized. Apart from analgesics the only treatment that is necessary is a mild diuretic, such as chlorthalidone (Hygroton) 50 mg, daily by mouth. It is important to monitor the patient's progress carefully and then to watch out for the onset of heart failure and pericarditis in particular. A repeat e.c.g. should be taken after a week and by this time the patient should be able to walk freely about the house on one level. If possible, it is best for patients to avoid using stairs more than once a day for at least three weeks and for this time should be confined to the house. If there are no complications the aim should be to return to normal activities within five or six weeks.

Medium and longer term complications of myocardial infarction

On the whole the prognosis for elderly people who have had a myocardial infarct is good, but there are some longer term complications that may adversely affect the outcome. The most important complication of myocardial infarction is the development of cardiac failure. Heart failure occurs quite frequently in the immediate post-infarction phase and does not affect the prognosis. However, when it occurs after a week or later it suggests a poor prognosis. This is presumably a reflection of extensive muscle damage, or it may be associated with papillary muscle dysfunction and consequent mitral valvular incompetence. In the older age group there is little that can be done about this except to treat the heart failure as it occurs with adequate diuretics.

Cardiac failure

Cardiac dysrhythmias frequently occur in the immediate post-infarction stage (see Chapter 3) and this is an indication for hospital admission. Major ventricular ectopic dysrhythmias may occur later, and we know that in younger patients this occurrence is associated with a poor prognosis and may cause sudden death. There is no reason to believe that the situation is any different in the elderly and these arrhythmias should be accurately identified and treated (see Chapter 3).

Cardiac dysrhythmias

Ventricular aneurysm probably occurs much more frequently than is generally recognized and this is a serious cause of heart failure and indicates a poor prognosis. In younger patients surgical correction is possible, but in the elderly this is not practicable. The diagnosis is confirmed by feeling a double apical impulse, by persistent S–T segment elevation on the e.c.g. and the X-ray findings of a boot-shaped heart or a bulge on the left ventricular outline which on screening pulsates paradoxically.

Ventricular aneurysm

Mural left ventricular thrombus formation may occur either in ventricular aneurysm or after extensive infarction and this may result in embolism into a major artery. The commonest sites are the carotid arteries and their branches and occasionally a 'saddle embolus' may lodge in the lower part of the aorta and block the iliac arteries. This results in absent femoral artery pulsation, and, if it is diagnosed quickly, is amenable to surgical removal. The patient should subsequently be put on longterm anticoagulant therapy and this is probably the only indication for these drugs after myocardial infarction.

Mural thrombus

Measured high blood pressure

There is considerable debate about what constitutes hypertension in the elderly and whether or not it should be treated. What is certain, however, is that malignant hypertension is excessively rare over the age of 70 years and is unlikely to be seen by a family doctor in a lifetime of practice.

It is well recognized that both systolic and diastolic blood pressures rise with age, although the rise tails off over the age of 70 years (Figure 2.4). In various studies of blood pressure measurements in the elderly a wide variation has been found. For example, in one large series of patients without obvious heart disease the middle 89% range included systolic blood pressures of up to 190 mmHg for men and over 200 mmHg for women; the same range for diastolic pressure went up to about 105 mmHg for men and 110 mmHg for women. One of the difficulties in this subject is the probable inaccuracy in the sphygmomanometer readings. In old people with arteriosclerotic brachial arteries it is unlikely that the intra-arterial pressure

Wide variation in 'normal' blood pressures

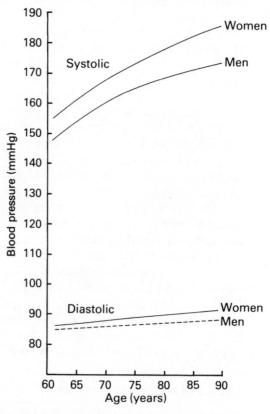

Rise in blood pressure with age in healthy subjects (From Anderson and Cowan, *Clin. Sci.*, 1959 with permission)

Figure 2.4

Difficulty of measuring true blood pressure

will correspond with the sphygmomanometer reading. Similarly the circumference of the arm and its muscularity have a considerable bearing on the blood pressure reading and should be corrected for – a fact that has been ignored in previous investigation of blood pressure. In patients with atrial fibrillation it is often very difficult to detect the diastolic end point at all and then the Korotkov phase 4 reading should be recorded.

Correlation with organ changes and heart disease

The correlation of raised blood pressure of long standing in old people with target organ changes such as left ventricular hypertrophy (Figure 2.5), retinal artery changes and renal impairment and proteinuria is poor and indeed several workers have found no increased mortality in the presence of either raised systolic or diastolic blood pressures (Figure 2.6). On the other hand the Framingham study suggested that a raised systolic blood pressure was associated with an increased mortality rate from ischaemic heart disease in the elderly (Figure 2.7).

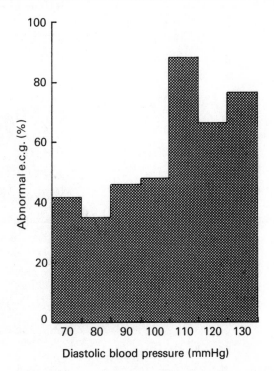

Figure 2.5

Incidence of abnormal e.c.g.s. with diastolic blood pressure (From Martin and Millard, *Age and Ageing*, 1973 with permission)

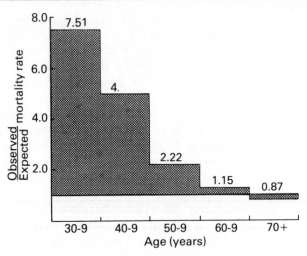

Observed/respected mortality at various ages (From Fry, *Common Diseases*, 1979, MTP Press with permission)

Figure 2.6

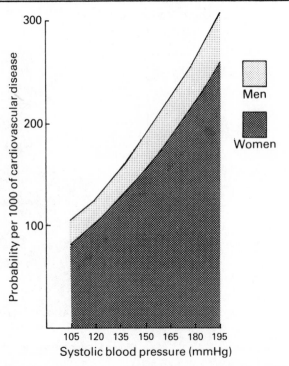

Probability of cardiovascular disease in 8 years in 70-year-olds according to a systolic blood pressure (Framingham Study, 1972)

Figure 2.7

Indications for treating measured high blood pressure

Although true hypertension is an unusual cause of heart failure in the elderly it is the main indication for treating the blood pressure when there is no other obvious cause, but it must be remembered that heart failure itself may sometimes result in an increase in the blood pressure. Thus it is important to record several resting blood pressure measurements, both lying and standing, before considering treatment. It is very unlikely that a systolic pressure of greater than 200 mmHg and a diastolic pressure of less than 110 mmHg will contribute significantly to the onset of heart failure and pressures below this require no more than diuretic therapy. If the retinal fundi are normal it is unlikely that the blood pressure requires treatment whatever the level.

A raised blood pressure may be found on routine examination and if this is greater than 200/110 and associated with retinal artery changes and left ventricular hypertrophy on the e.c.g. then it is wise to consider treatment if repeated blood pressure measurements are also high.

When not to treat measured high blood pressure

Contra-
indications

There are several contraindications to the treatment of blood pressure. It is essential to measure the pressure in both the lying and standing positions and if there is a drop of greater than 20 mmHg in the systolic pressure then treatment is likely to cause serious postural hypotension.

Stroke

There is good evidence to show that patients who have had a stroke or suffer from dementia will not be helped by a reduction in blood pressure and in some cases will be made considerably worse. However high the manometric reading may be, it should be ignored – in fact it may well be wiser not to measure the blood pressure at all! Once target organ damage has occurred treatment will usually make the situation worse and the same rule applies to progressive renal impairment.

Investigation and the choice of anti-hypertensive treatment

General
assessment

If the physician decides, having noted the above comments, to reduce a patient's blood pressure, he should make a general assessment of the patient. Obesity should be treated and may result in a significant reduction in pressure. Renal function should be assessed and urinalysis performed. An accurate assessment of the retinal fundi should be made and the e.c.g. performed. A chest X-ray to show the heart clearly must be taken. It is wise to estimate the fasting and 2-hour postprandial blood sugars to exclude diabetes and the uric acid and cholesterol levels in the blood should be checked.

Drug treatment should start with a thiazide diuretic, such as cyclopenthiazide, (Navidrex) or bendrofluazide (Neo-Naclex) with a potassium supplement, provided there is no evidence of diabetes. This treatment usually results in a useful reduction in pressure. If further treatment is required a beta-blocking agent such as propranolol (Inderal) 10 mg, Oxprenolol (Trasicor) 40 mg three times a day should be used. Both these agents are now available in a slow-release form and enable once daily dosage, which is sometimes an important consideration in the elderly. There are many beta-blocking agents available and there is little practical evidence that one is better than another for the control of blood pressure. The major contraindication to the use of these drugs is the presence of chronic obstructive airways disease. In the event of further drug treatment being necessary, methyldopa, prazosin or bethanidine may be used. The main object of treatment is to cause a very gentle lowering of the blood pressure since any sharp falls in pressure will cause severe side-effects and may even result in a stroke (Table 2.2).

Table 2.2   Antihypertensive regime for the elderly

	Comments
1. Diuretic	
Benzothiadiazines	Glucose intolerance
(hydrochlorothiazide, bendro-	Potassium loss
fluazide)	Uric acid retention
Triamterene	Less powerful than thiazides
	Potassium sparing
2. Beta-adrenoreceptor antagonists	Bradycardia
	Glucose intolerance
(a) Lipid soluble	
(propranolol, oxprenolol)	Small doses required in liver insufficiency
(b) Water soluble	
(acebutalol, atenolol, sotalol)	High blood levels in renal dysfunction
3. Other agents (If diuretics and beta-blockers unsatisfactory or contraindicated	
(a) Methyldopa	Postural hypotension
	Rarely causes haemolytic anaemia

Table 2.2 (Continued)

(b) Prazosin	Postural hypotension
	Powerful hypotensive agent
(c) Hydrallazine	Reflex tachycardia
	Rarely produces SLE syndrome

Valvular heart disease

Rheumatic and congenital disease

One still sees rheumatic heart disease in the elderly and even, occasionally, congenital heart disease. With the introduction of powerful diuretic agents and the greater success of cardiac surgery in the last two decades many patients with significant rheumatic valvular disease may live to a great age. These patients are generally, but not always, already under the care of a heart specialist in hospital and their management is not likely to cause problems for the family doctor, except for the treatment of intercurrent chest infections and heart failure. There are, however, some mild degrees of rheumatic valve disease that have gone unrecognized before and present as a new problem for the general practitioner. It is thus always important to bear this in mind when seeing a new patient with heart failure and a murmur.

Degenerative

Syphilis

Bacterial endocarditis

The great majority of valvular disease in the elderly is a result of degenerative change in either the aortic or, more commonly, the mitral valve. The aortic valve may suffer from calcium deposition upon it. This usually results in sclerosis of the valve, but there may be a degree of stenosis or incompetence. Occasionally the aortic valve may be the site of tertiary syphilitic infection, which causes destruction of the valve cusps. This condition is usually associated with other signs of the disease, especially tabes dorsalis or dementia. It is always essential to check the serological tests for syphilis. Apart from rheumatic involvement the aortic valve may also be damaged by bacterial endocarditis and this condition is now known to affect a valve that has any abnormality, such as calcium deposition upon it.

Mucoid degeneration

It is now increasingly recognized that the mitral valve is frequently the cause of murmurs in the elderly. Apart from rheumatic valvular stenosis and incompetence, the usual cause of mitral valve disease in the elderly is mucoid degeneration. The valve, however, may also be affected by papillary muscle damage that occurs after myocardial infarction. Both these last two disorders cause prolapsing of the posterior cusp of the valve and consequent incompetence. Calcification of the mitral valve may also occur and sometimes this extends below the cusps and interferes with blood flow.

Clinical features of senile mitral incompetence

This is probably one of the commonest valvular lesions seen in old people and is frequently mistaken for aortic sclerosis or stenosis. The murmur is quite different from aortic murmurs and also differs from the classical rheumatic mitral incompetence, in that the murmur does not occupy the whole of systole and may, in fact, occur quite late in systole. It is frequently preceded by an ejection click. The murmur is often rough and may be very loud. It is also usually widely radiated both to the left axilla and over the whole of the praecordium. The left ventricle may be enlarged and this may be seen both on the chest X-ray and the electrocardiogram.

Clinical features of aortic valve disease

Aortic sclerosis

A systolic murmur in the aortic area radiating up into the neck should alert one to the diagnosis of aortic sclerosis. The absence of any pulse wave abnormalities at the wrist and an aortic systolic thrill almost certainly confirm the diagnosis. Sometimes the rigid valve may also leak a little and there may be a short, soft, early diastolic murmur as well. These patients often have evidence of sclerotic vessels elsewhere and calcification in other parts of the thoracic and abdominal aorta. The electrocardiogram will not show any evidence of left ventricular hypertrophy, unless there is another cause for it. The patient will not suffer any symptoms from the sclerosis of the valve and no action need be taken.

Aortic stenosis

This lesion is quite a different matter. Patients may well suffer symptoms such as angina, fainting attacks and heart failure. The physical signs are also different; there is a slow-rising radial pulse, a small pulse pressure, a systolic thrill and loud aortic murmur with wide radiation. The left ventricle is enlarged clinically and electrocardiographically. On the chest X-ray the left ventricle is dilated and there may be calcification in the valve as well as in the aorta. If the symptoms are severe it is worth considering operative replacement of the valve and whatever the age of the patient, it is worth referring him to the hospital specialist if his general health and mental state are good. Heart failure carries a poor prognosis in aortic stenosis and if any surgical procedures are contemplated, action must be taken quickly.

Aortic incompetence

This may be associated with either sclerosis or stenosis of the valve, but in the former is rarely of any great significance. Severe degrees of aortic regurgitation occur with tertiary syphilitic disease or can be due to a rupture of a valve cusp. Rheumatic heart disease may have damaged the valve and bacterial endocarditis may also further damage it (see below). Incompetence may lead to angina and heart failure if it is severe and treatment is the same as for aortic stenosis. Clinically there is a waterhammer or collapsing pulse and a large pulse pressure. There is a loud aortic diastolic murmur immediately following the accentuated aortic second heart sound. The e.c.g. confirms left ventricular hypertrophy, as does the chest X-ray, which also may show calcification of the ascending part of the aorta if there is syphilitic disease. It is always wise to do the serological tests for syphilis in this condition. Tertiary syphilis should be treated with a full 10 day course of intramuscular penicillin.

Bacterial endocarditis

This is a condition that has changed in character over the last few decades. It is usually rather more acute than the classical description of subacute bacterial endocarditis that was seen until the 1950s. It is a disease that is not uncommonly seen in the elderly and must always be considered in a patient with a fever and changing murmurs. The causative organism is frequently a staphylococcus or a coliform rather than *Streptococcus viridans*, and usually arises from the gut, urinary tract or gall bladder. It is now well recognized that these organisms may affect any damaged valve rather than occurring in those patients who have had rheumatic heart disease.

The disease is serious and there is still a significant mortality if the diagnosis is not made early. The onset may be insidious but the history is more likely to be of short duration. The cardinal features are fever, heart murmurs and systemic embolism. The emboli are most frequently seen in the kidneys, producing microscopic haematuria, the brain, causing confusion and focal neurological signs and the skin, which may result in Osler's nodes, petechiae and splinter haemorrhages. Sometimes the presenting feature may be heart failure due to damage of the aortic valve cusps. It is no use waiting for the full-blown classical clinical picture of endocarditis to appear before suspecting the disease, because by the time that clubbing of fingers and the other signs described above are seen the disease will be well advanced and the prognosis is extremely poor. There is a mortality rate of up to 70% in the elderly. The certain evidence of a septicaemia, together with heart murmurs, is sufficient to diagnose endocarditis and vigorous treatment at this stage will reduce the mortality rate to near zero.

It is essential to take several blood cultures before giving antibiotics. It is not practicable to treat the patient at home and early hospital admission should be sought. The correct treatment is to give a full six weeks course of the appropriate antibiotic, having identified the causative organism and its sensitivity to drugs. Once the blood cultures have been taken it is reasonable to start treatment with a parenteral broad spectrum antibiotic such as amoxycillin or a cephalosporin drug and these can be changed in the light of the bacteriological report.

Heart failure

Heart failure is one of the commonest problems that the family doctor will encounter in his elderly patients. Heart failure may be purely left-sided or right-sided, or more frequently congestive. The classical signs of heart failure are generally well recognized, but despite this there is frequently some delay in making the diagnosis in old people. It is essential to recognize that heart failure is a symptom and not a disease and there must always be some reason for it to occur. It is not sufficient merely to give diuretic agents, because unless the causative condition is recognized and treated the heart failure will recur.

Importance of diagnosis of underlying cause

Left ventricular failure

This condition is sometimes very difficult to identify. The symptoms arise because of failure of the left ventricle to cope with the blood inflow from the pulmonary veins, with resultant pulmonary congestion. The earliest symptoms may be purely

Dyspnoea

36

dyspnoea on exertion, but often the presenting symptom of left heart failure is paroxysmal nocturnal dyspnoea. Sudden onset of dyspnoea at night always indicates left heart failure and these patients cannot lie flat. Unless there is a history of chronic lung disease, the sudden onset of dyspnoea in the elderly always suggests left ventricular failure. Since left-sided failure is usually a self-limiting condition some patients may have had several attacks of nocturnal dyspnoea before they call the doctor, and direct questioning about their sleeping habits and the number of pillows used is important.

Gallop rhythm Auscultation of the heart may show evidence of left ventricular enlargement, there may be a murmur and there is a fourth heart sound. The lung bases will be full of crepitations.

It is essential to diagnose the cause of left heart failure and very often this is due to cardiac dysrhythmia, most commonly atrial fibrillation. The pulse may give evidence of this and may be rapid and regular or irregular. Auscultation of the

Atrial fibrillation heart may confirm atrial fibrillation or paroxysmal tachycardia and the definitive diagnosis is made from the e.c.g. (see

Myocardial infarction Chapter 3). Other common causes of left heart failure are myocardial infarction and mitral incompetence or aortic stenosis or incompetence (see above).

Treatment

The treatment of left ventricular failure from whatever cause is with intravenous diamorphine or morphine, aminophylline and frusemide 40–80 mg. Any cardiac dysrhythmia should be identified and treated appropriately (see Chapter 3). If these measures are not immediately successful, cuffing of the limbs should be practised. There is no indication to lower the blood pressure at this stage, even if hypertension may be the cause of the failure; the above measures should be quite sufficient and allow consideration and assessment of the blood pressure status at leisure (see above).

Congestive cardiac failure

Continued back pressure on the pulmonary circulation from a failing left ventricle will ultimately lead to right ventricular failure and the combination results in congestive heart failure. The acute severe dyspnoea disappears and is replaced by

Oedema oedema, chronic dyspnoea and lethargy. The oedema is dependent and usually leads to swollen legs, but if the patient is lying in bed there will be a sacral pad of oedema. Old people may

37

tolerate advanced degrees of congestive heart failure and the oedema may be gross and, not uncommonly, may spread to involve the whole leg and even the trunk. Clinical examination will show an elevation of the jugular venous pressure and it is a useful sign that many modern doctors have lost the habit of demonstrating. There may also be a pleural effusion, this is usually bilateral, but may be unilateral and is more common on the right than the left. The liver is usually palpable and tender and there may be ascites in advanced cases. Right sided heart failure, caused by chronic lung disease and mitral stenosis, will produce a similar picture and can be distinguished from congestive heart failure by the history and the electrocardiogram, which shows evidence of right ventricular hypertrophy and large and abnormally shaped P waves (P mitrale and P pulmonale). The diagnosis of right ventricular hypertrophy on the e.c.g. is often very difficult owing to the natural dominance of the left ventricular repolarization.

Treatment

The treatment of congestive heart failure is with diuretic agents and with correction of the underlying cause, as far as this is possible. There is little evidence that digoxin is of any great value unless there is atrial fibrillation and this is discussed more fully in Chapter 3. There is little difference in the treatment with diuretic agents in the elderly compared with that in younger patients. The elderly may need massive doses of diuretics if the failure is resistant to normal doses and the family doctor should not be afraid of using large doses of powerful diuretic drugs, such as frusemide (Lasix), bumetamide (Burinex) or ethacrynic acid (Edecrin), if the clinical situation demands it. Potassium supplementation should be given, although recent evidence has shown that this is not so critical as was thought a year or so ago, if the patient is taking a normal diet. Once the failure is under control it will be possible to reduce the dose of these drugs and possibly to change to other diuretics, such as thiazide, triamterene or amiloride. It is important to realize that all diuretic agents interfere with glucose metabolism and may upset diabetic control or even precipitate the diabetic state. The use of diuretics is more fully discussed in Chapter 10.

The differential diagnosis of swollen legs

Gravitation   The commonest cause of swollen legs in an old person is dependent oedema due to gravitation and varicose veins. Because of

38

their natural tendency to sit around, elderly people often get swelling of their legs, without any evidence of heart disease. Gravitational oedema is a phenomenon that is now well-recognized in young fit people as a result of sitting immobile for long periods in aeroplanes and longdistance buses, and the situation is exactly the same in the elderly who spend long periods sitting in a chair in front of the fire or the television set. Patients with varicose veins suffer a similar problem with rather less causal stress. Diuretic drugs are absolutely useless in this situation and the problem is usually easily solved if general advice is given about mobility and leg exercises. If there is chronic venous obstruction elastic stockings will help greatly. Gravitational oedema is rarely caused by hypoproteinaemia, whether this is the result of dietary insufficiency, protein loss or liver failure. These conditions are not usually difficult to diagnose, but should always be borne in mind in cases of resistant oedema.

Elastic stockings

Disorders of the cardiovascular system (II)

IRREGULARITIES OF THE PULSE: DISORDERS OF CARDIAC RHYTHM AND CONDUCTION AND PACEMAKERS

The incidence of irregularities of the pulse – The conducting system of the heart – Disorders of the conducting system – Symptoms of cardiac arrhythmias – Methods of assessing irregularities of the pulse – Some of more common arrhythmias in the elderly – Ectopic beats – Tachycardias – Disorders of conduction – Cardiac pacemakers

Electrocardiographic diagnosis is becoming more important for general practitioners, since these problems are common in the elderly, there are now many effective drugs available to treat these arrhythmias and many family doctors have electrocardiographs and are thus in a good position to identify and treat disorders of cardiac rhythm and conduction in the home.

The successful introduction of artificial cardiac pacemakers has revolutionized the management of diseases of the conducting system and it is important for the family doctor to have a working knowledge of the indications for pacemaker insertion and to understand something of the problems that may arise in his patients with these generators at home.

The incidence of irregularities of the pulse

Effect of age Cardiac arrhythmias occur at all ages, but their incidence rises markedly with increasing age. In the elderly there is the extra problem of the degenerative changes that appear in the conducting system, resulting in heart block and sinus node disease.

41

Ventricular
ectopic beats

In healthy old people at home the family physician can expect that 70% will have ventricular ectopic beats (see Table 3.1), but in only 12–15% are these of such a frequency or multifocal in origin such as to suggest that they are of clinical significance.

Table 3.1 Incidence of ventricular arrhythmias in healthy people at home aged 75 years and over

Minor	Isolated ventricular extrasystoles (<10/h)	42%
	Moderate ventricular extrasystoles (10–100/h)	14%
Major	Frequent ventricular extrasystoles (>100/h)	12%
	Multiform ventricular extrasystoles	22%
	Ventricular bigeminy	9%
	Salvoes of ventricular extrasystoles	2%
	Paroxysmal ventricular tachycardia	4%

Supraventricular
ectopic beats

Supraventricular ectopic beats are also common and occur in over 30% of healthy persons but these too may have no prognostic significance. Episodes of supraventricular tachycardia may occur in about 4% of the elderly if they are monitored for a 24 hour period, but atrial fibrillation occurs in 10% of these patients.

Atrial
fibrillation

Atrial fibrillation may be established or paroxysmal. Sinus bradycardia of significant degree probably occurs in about 10% of the elderly and reflects disease of the sinus node. The concept of sinus node disease is important as far as the elderly are concerned and a whole section will be devoted to this topic.

Table 3.2 Incidence of arrhythmias in the over 70s

Atrial fibrillation*	11%
Ventricular ectopics* (< 100/h)	56%
Frequent ventricular ectopics† (> 100/h)	12%
Multifocal ventricular ectopics†	22%
Runs of ventricular ectopics†	
Ventricular tachycardia †	9%
Complete heart block †	1%

*Minor arrhythmias
†Major arrhythmias (Lown's criteria)
(These figures are approximate values)

The conducting system of the heart

Many cells throughout the heart have the ability to discharge electrical impulses and this inherent discharge is known as 'automaticity'. The sino-atrial (SA) node has the highest degree of automaticity and is normally the cardiac pacemaker. The SA node discharge rate is under the influence of the vagus (slowing) and sympathetic (accelerating) nerves and is also affected by other stimuli such as thyroxine and toxins. From the SA node impulses pass through the atrial walls to the atrioventricular (AV) node and from thence into the His–Purkinje system. The bundle of His starts in the AV node (see diagram) and branches into the left and right bundles. The left bundle further subdivides into the anterior and posterior fascicles. The bundles of His terminate in the Purkinje fibres that lie in the ventricular walls.

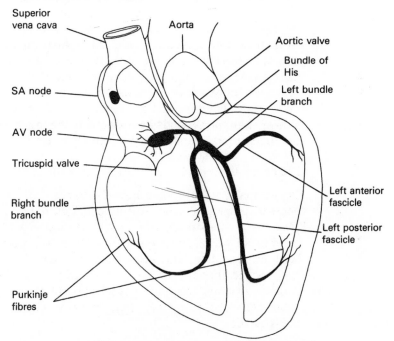

The normal conducting system of the heart

Disorders of the conducting system

The normal processes of heart rhythm control in the elderly may become damaged intermittently or permanently in ischaemic heart disease. However, there are a number of other causes of conduction tissue disease and these include primary myocardial disease such as Lenegre's and Lev's syndromes, cardiomyopathy, especially alcoholic and beri-beri in the elderly, infiltrative diseases, such as senile cardiac amyloidosis and neoplasm, and metabolic disturbances such as hypolalaemia and hypercalcaemia. Drugs may cause conduction tissue disturbances, with digitalis as the most frequent offender, but the beta-blocking drugs and the other anti-arrhythmic agents may have unwanted effects on the heart.

Escape beats and extrasystoles may be a sign of conduction tissue disease and are particularly important since they may initiate ectopic rhythms that may be dangerous and sometimes fatal.

Escape beats

The conducting system may be diseased at any point. If the SA node is involved the condition is known as 'sino-atrial disease'. The normal dominant cardiac pacemaker then fails and an 'escape beat' or 'escape rhythm' may intervene. There are many potential pacemaker cells throughout the atria, AV node and the ventricles and any of these may take up the role of the pacemaker when the protective influence of the SA node is removed; for example, nodal escape beats or even nodal rhythm may occur. The inherent automaticity of these cells is always slower than the SA node and generally the lower down the conducting system the slower the rate of automaticity.

Extrasystoles

Occasionally the potential discharge of a subsidiary pacemaker may be prematurely precipitated by a sinus beat. There is a constant coupling interval; that is a constant relationship of all unifocal ectopic beats to the preceding sinus beat. Extrasystoles may arise from any part of the heart. They may occur haphazardly or regularly and they may be multifocal when they arise from several sites. By definition three consecutive ectopic beats constitutes an extrasystolic tachycardia.

Heart block

This generally refers to conduction block at the AV node. But block also occurs commonly in the bundles of His. Generally one or other of the main right or left bundles is obstructed, but more recently it has been realized that only one of the anterior or posterior fascicles of the left bundle--may be blocked (hemiblock) either alone or more significantly in association with right bundle branch block. Heart block and bundle branch block are discussed in more detail below.

Symptoms of cardiac arrhythmias

Many patients have no symptoms as a result of disturbances of cardiac rhythm and even major disorders such as rapid supraventricular tachycardia or intermittent complete heart block may cause a patient no trouble. On the other hand the elderly may frequently complain of palpitations or giddiness when there is no demonstrable cardiac abnormality. The poor correlation between patient symptoms and demonstrable rhythm disturbances is a major problem for the investigating physician. The correct interpretation of the electrocardiogram (e.c.g.) is absolutely fundamental since relatively minor abnormalities, such as left anterior hemiblock (LAH) or non-conducted atrial bigeminy, may go unnoticed and yet reflect serious disease of the conducting system; if the family physician is in any doubt as to the interpretation of the e.c.g. he should refer it to a specialist in the field.

Poor correlation between symptoms and disturbance

In distinction from younger patients, disturbances of the heart rhythm in the elderly frequently give rise to symptoms, presumably due to co-existent cerebrovascular disease, where any transient reduction in cardiac output may critically affect normal cerebration. Thus the most frequent symptoms of rhythm disturbances in the elderly are those of disordered brain function. Giddiness and falling are common, but on the other hand there are many other causes of these symptoms (see Chapter 6) and these must be excluded. Syncopal attacks and confusional states are often the result of cardiac disease, but again there are many other causes that have to be considered. Epileptic fits and strokes may be caused by rhythm changes, and in these patients it is essential to consider a cardiac cause. Angina may be precipitated by either very rapid or slow heart rates in the absence of obvious ischaemic heart disease, and correct treatment is very gratifying. Left ventricular failure may also be the presenting symptom of cardiac arrhythmias, especially of rapid atrial fibrillation.

Disordered brain function

Epileptic fits and strokes

Angina

Left ventricular failure

Methods of assessing irregularities of the pulse

Pulse Palpation of the radial pulse will usually produce evidence of cardiac arrhythmias, but on occasions it will be very difficult to detect slow atrial fibrillation unless the cardiac apex is examined at the same time. Non-conducted atrial premature beats cannot be detected from examination of the radial pulse or auscultation of the heart. Ventricular ectopic beats are

45

usually detected at the wrist by a pause in the pulse, as they frequently do not give rise to effective ventricular contraction, but they cannot usually be distinguished from sino-atrial block or sinus node arrest. Sinus bradycardia may be profoundly slow with sinus rates as low as 20 beats per minute and it is almost impossible to distinguish this from heart block or non-conducted atrial bigeminy without reading an electrocardiogram (e.c.g.).

Electrocardio-
gram
The e.c.g. is the fundamental investigation in interpreting disorders of cardiac rhythm and most of the chapter is devoted to this subject. There are, however, situations where the 12-lead resting e.c.g. is inadequate for detecting cardiac arrhythmias and there are two situations when other techniques are required. After myocardial infarction it may be necessary to continuously monitor the heart and this is done by means of an oscilloscope; the indications for this in the elderly are discussed in Chapter 2.

The other method of investigating rhythm disorders is by means of ambulatory cardiac monitoring or dynamic electrocardiography (d.c.g.). This technique is performed using a battery-powered reel-to-reel tape recorder attached by leads to the patient's chest and can be performed in the home. Most recorders are worn for 24 hours and do not significantly interfere with the patient's activities. The tape is then removed and analysed by a computerized play-back machine at rates of up to 120 times real time. It is then possible to identify the number and type of any ectopic beats, the frequency and duration of any ectopic tachycardia, monitor the sinus rate and assess any degree of heart block. Most recorders have a digital 'events' timing clock and thus it is possible to correlate the symptoms of which the patient complains with the d.c.g. tracing. The special value of the d.c.g. in the elderly is in the investigation of fits, faints and falls (see Chapter 6) where the cause may be a disturbance of cardiac output due to an arrhythmia or heart block. Dynamic electrocardiography may also be used in the assessment of pacemaker performance and also in an evaluation of the significance of ectopic beats after myocardial infarction and their response to treatment.

Some of the more common arrhythmias in the elderly

Cardiac arrhythmias are frequent in the elderly and their interpretation and management can often be undertaken by the family physician. Further investigation is often necessary in a specialist department in hospital but the family doctor is often in a good position to diagnose an arrhythmia since he will see the patient in his normal environment where most of these problems occur and this is especially important in the elderly as many of these arrhythmias are intermittent.

Ectopic beats

These may arise from any part of the heart, but are most frequently atrial, junctional (arising from the AV node) or ventricular.

Atrial ectopic beats

The P wave is premature and usually misshapen. The QRS complex is nearly always normal, but rarely there may be aberrated conduction with a bizarre and widened QRS complex. There is always a compensatory pause following the ectopic beat which is longer than the normal sinus cycle.

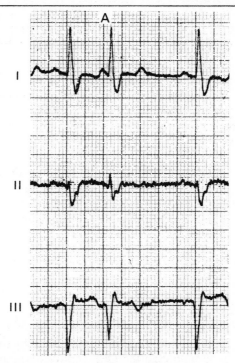

Figure 3.1   Atrial ectopic beat (A) with normal conduction

47

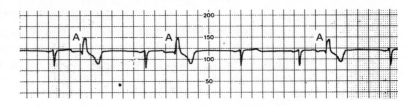

Figure 3.2 Atrial ectopic beat (A) with aberrated conduction·

Occasionally atrial ectopic beats may occur in a bigeminal rhythm and very often these are not conducted through the AV node as they fall in its refractory period. This condition can only be diagnosed by means of an e.c.g. and is easily mistaken for sinus bradycardia or even heart block.

Atrial ectopic beats are probably of no clinical significance except that they may occasionally initiate atrial fibrillation. They require no treatment unless they occur in a bigeminal rhythm when they usually respond very well to the

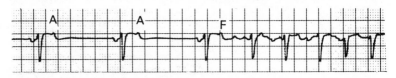

Non-conducted atrial premature beats masquerading as sinus brady cardia (A) and initiating atrial fibrillation (F)

Figure 3.3

administration of oral disopyramide (Rythmodan) in divided doses of 300–600 mg per day. Since atrial bigeminy is often associated with sino-atrial disease (see below) disopyramide will increase the normal sinus rate and depress ectopic atrial activity.

Junctional ectopic beats

The premature beat is characterized by an abnormal and often inverted P wave which may be immediately preceding, buried in or following the QRS complex which is itself almost normal The ectopic beat is followed by a compensatory pause.

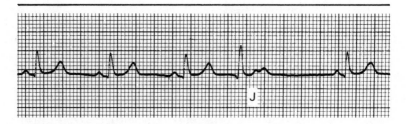

Figure 3.4

Junctional ectopic beat (J)

Ventricular ectopic beats

These premature beats show no P wave normally and the QRS complex is bizarre and widened as in a bundle branch block pattern (see below). These ectopic beats may arise from different foci (multifocal) and the QRS pattern will vary in the same e.c.g. lead.

If ventricular ectopic beats are isolated and occur at a frequency of less than 100 per hour as counted on a d.c.g. record-

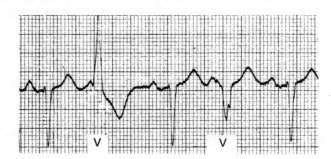

Figure 3.5

Multifocal ventricular ectopic beats (V)

ing then they are probably of no significance. However, if they are multifocal or occur in pairs or in a bigeminal rhythm they are of clinical significance, especially after a myocardial infarction and should be treated. Disopyramide, mexiletine and verapamil are usually effective in controlling these ectopics.

Significance of ectopic beats

The main importance of recognizing ectopic beats is that they may predispose to other more significant arrhythmias and may be a sign of digitalis overdosage or electrolyte disturbance.

49

Tachycardias

Atrial fibrillation

This is one of the commonest tachycardias occurring in the elderly. It may be intermittent or established and probably always starts off by being intermittent. It is a feature of sino-atrial disease (see below) and a frequent occurrence after myocardial infarction. Intermittent atrial fibrillation is almost always associated with a rapid ventricular rate and may well cause left ventricular failure. Established atrial fibrillation is associated with a well controlled ventricular rate in about half the patients and needs no treatment unless there is an associat-

Thyro- ed intercurrent infection or thyrotoxicosis. It is worth remem-
toxicosis bering that thyrotoxicosis is always associated with atrial fibrillation, established or intermittent, in patients over 70 years. The clinical features of atrial fibrillation are an ir-regularly irregular heart action and the e.c.g. shows the absence of normal P waves, which are replaced with 'f' waves which occur at a rate of between 400 and 600 per minute. It has been suggested that coarse 'f' waves occur in patients whose atrial fibrillation is of recent onset and sometimes they may be mistaken for 'F' waves of atrial flutter (see below). The QRS complexes are usually normal in width, but are irregular in time and in form.

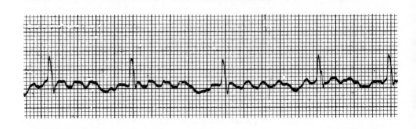

Atrial fibrillation (coarse)

Figure 3.6

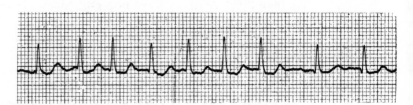

Atrial fibrillation

Figure 3.7

Treatment

The treatment of atrial fibrillation is either with digoxin alone, or, as recent evidence would suggest, with a combination of digoxin and beta blocker in small doses. Beta blockade is better avoided if there is heart failure or a history of airways obstruction, but in a few instances where the heart failure is due to the tachycardia and is uncontrolled with digoxin alone it is reasonable to give beta blockers as well. Many of these patients will have some degree of heart failure and a diuretic drug will need to be given in combination with the other drugs. The dose of digitalis will have to be carefully monitored and elderly patients cannot tolerate this drug very well (see Chapter 10). There is no indication to try and convert atrial fibrillation in the elderly to sinus rhythm by direct current countershock.

Atrial flutter

This is not a common arrhythmia in the elderly. The atrial rate is about 300 per minute and there is always a degree of AV nodal block, which is usually fixed as 3:1 or 4:1. Some patients can tolerate atrial flutter very well when the ventricular rate is about 80 per minute and the degree of AV block is 4:1 or 5:1 and no treatment is necessary. The diagnosis is made from the e.c.g. which shows the presence of 'F' waves at the rate of about 300 per minute. The QRS complex is normal unless there is associated bundle branch block.

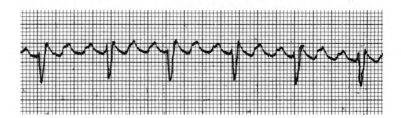

Figure 3.8

Atrial flutter with 3:1 AV nodal block

Treatment

If the ventricular rate is rapid the degree of AV block can be increased by giving digitalis which slows the ventricular rate. It may be preferable to refer patients with atrial flutter to a hospital where the arrhythmia can be abolished by means of direct current countershock.

Supraventricular tachycardia (SVT)

This is seen much less commonly in the elderly than in younger patients. The focus for the tachycardia may lie in the atria or the AV node and from a practical point of view the distinction is academic. SVT may be associated with myocardial infarction and also occurs frequently in the short P–R interval syndromes (Lown–Ganong–Levine and Wolff–Parkinson–White). Paroxysmal SVT also occurs in patients with sino-atrial disease and in some of these may be associated with periods of severe bradycardia (bradycardia–tachycardia syndrome). The importance of this condition in the elderly is that it is frequently associated with faints and falls because of the sudden changes in cardiac output and is often very difficult to diagnose without using ambulatory monitoring. The diagnosis is made from the e.c.g., where the P waves may not easily be seen or are buried in the normal shaped QRS complexes. The heart rate is between 160 and 220 per minute and there may be abnormal ST segments and T waves. Sometimes SVT may be associated with a bundle branch block and it is then difficult to differentiate from paroxysmal ventricular tachycardia.

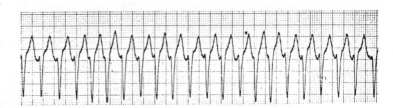

Figure 3.9 Supraventricular tachycardia

Treatment

It is always worth trying the effect of carotid sinus massage in SVT as this may terminate the event, but it must be done under e.c.g. control. Very often in the elderly, carotid sinus massage is ineffective and then it is worth trying the effect of intravenous practolol or disopyramide. All these manoeuvres must be monitored on the e.c.g. and it may be more convenient to send the patient to hospital where he may be monitored by an oscilloscope. The bradycardia–tachycardia syndrome is discussed further under the section on sino-atrial disease.

Ventricular tachycardia

This rhythm is usually only seen after myocardial infarction or on ambulatory d.c.g. tapes as a transient feature. The rate is slower than in SVT and is usually between 150 and 200 per minute. The P waves are not seen and the QRS complexes are widened with abnormal T waves. Sometimes one may see ventricular flutter where the QRS complexes merge imperceptibly with the bizarre preceding T waves. The rate is usually fast and over 220 per minute.

Treatment

The treatment of ventricular tachycardia at home is with disopyramide or mexiletine, but this is a condition that is unlikely to be seen often in the home except in myocardial infarction when it is usually preceded by ventricular ectopic beats and which are an indication to refer the patient to hospital (see Chapter 2).

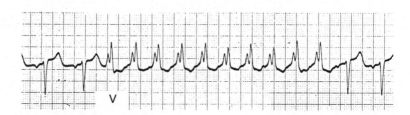

Figure 3.10 Ventricular tachycardia (V)

Ventricular fibrillation

This arrhythmia is only included for completeness, since it is a terminal event and will rarely be seen outside an intensive care unit. Ventricular activity is completely chaotic and unco-ordinated and there are no recognizable waveforms. It is often initiated by a ventricular ectopic beat coinciding with the preceding T wave (the R on T phenomenon).

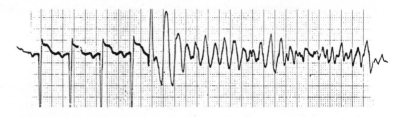

Figure 3.11 Ventricular fibrillation initiated by the R on T phenomenon

Disorders of conduction

Sino-atrial disease

This is an important and common problem in the elderly. It can be shown that with age there is a progressive diminution in the number of cells in the sinus node and this probably accounts for the failure of the SA node as the dominant pacemaker. The conditions associated with sino-atrial disease are listed in Table 3.3.

Table 3.3 Features of sino-atrial disease

Sinus bradycardia
Fixed sinus rate
SA block (sinus arrest)
Escape rhythm
Atrial fibrillation
Atrial flutter
Bradycardia–tachycardia syndrome

Sinus bradycardia

This is defined as a sinus rhythm below 60 beats per minute during waking hours, but will only cause problems if it is severe, with sinus rates well below 50 beats per minute. It is now recognized that severe sinus bradycardia may be as slow as 20 per minute. With these slow rates the cardiac output is critically reduced and patients will get angina and fainting attacks. Also under these circumstances subsidiary pacemakers may become manifest producing as an 'escape' beat or 'escape' rhythm such as idiojunctional or idioventricular rhythms.

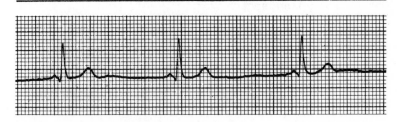

Figure 3.12

Sinus bradycardia (40 beats per minute) in a patient with faints

Fixed sinus rate

Some old people have an inability to change their sinus rate in response to stress and this feature may be due either to breakdown of the autonomic nervous system or the sinus node. In either event patients may get symptoms of dyspnoea on exertion or angina and many patients later develop more serious signs of conduction tissue disease.

SA block (sinus arrest)

This is quite a common occurrence in the elderly. SA block, where there is a failure of transmission of conduction between the SA node and the atria and sinus arrest, where the sinus node fails to discharge, are extremely difficult to distinguish electrocardiographically. The e.c.g. findings are of intermittently absent P waves and the P–P interval is about twice the length of normal. Usually the next beat after SA block is a sinus one, but there may be an escape beat arising from another focus. SA block frequently gives rise to symptoms.

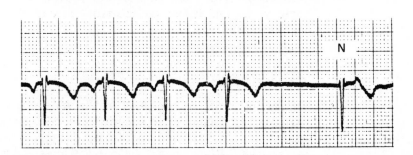

Figure 3.13

SA block followed by nodal escape beat (N)

55

Treatment

Occasionally SA block may be more prolonged and there is a longer period of cardiac arrest, which may well cause syncope. These patients should be treated with a cardiac pacemaker. Sometimes the escape beat may lead into an escape rhythm occurring from the same focus.

Atrial fibrillation and atrial flutter have been described above.

Bradycardia–tachycardia syndrome

This syndrome is an important feature of sino-atrial disease and, as its name implies, is characterized by reciprocating periods of bradycardia and tachycardia. The most frequent dysrhythmias are a combination of sinus bradycardia and atrial fibrillation, but sinus bradycardia may alternate with paroxysmal supraventricular tachycardia. This syndrome usually gives rise to major symptoms of giddiness and fainting and is characteristically difficult to identify by means of the 12 lead e.c.g. since the periods of dysrhythmia are usually fairly brief. If the condition is suspected, ambulatory cardiac monitoring is extremely helpful, but more than one 24 hour tape recording may be necessary.

Treatment

The treatment of the bradycardia–tachycardia syndrome with drugs is not very satisfactory because although it is possible to control the tachycardia with anti-arrhythmic agents these will not help the sinus bradycardia. Usually it is necessary to insert a permanent on-demand cardiac pacemaker. This does not always prevent the paroxysmal tachycardia and it may be necessary to give anti-arrhythmic agents as well.

Atrioventricular block

Conduction block at the level of the AV node is usually a feature of ischaemic or degenerative heart disease, but in the elderly is often caused by drugs, especially the digitalis derivatives. With rapid supraventricular tachycardias, especially atrial fibrillation, there is always a degree of AV block which constantly varies and results in an irregular heart rate. Atrioventricular block may be intermittent and is then only identified by longterm monitoring, but more usually it is established and is easily shown on the 12 lead e.c.g. All forms of AV block may be seen after acute myocardial infarction and this is a major indication for referral of the patient to an intensive care unit.

First degree AV block

This is characterized by a prolongation of the P−R interval beyond 0.22 s. Perhaps surprisingly it is not often seen in the elderly unless they are taking digitalis. It has been said that this conduction abnormality is benign, but if it is found in an old person who has not had a myocardial infarction or who is taking digitalis it may well be a premonitory sign of more sinister degrees of heart block and should not be ignored.

No symptoms arise from this abnormality and no treatment is necessary.

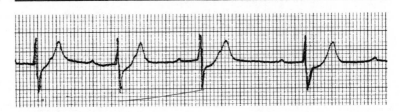

First degree AV block

Figure 3.14

Second degree AV block

The Wenckebach phenomenon (Mobitz type I block)

There is a progressive prolongation of the P−R interval and the sequence terminates in a blocked sinus beat (a P wave not followed by a QRS complex). These sequences are usually repeated and the varying A-V conduction ratios (3:2, 4:3, 5:4, etc.) result in an irregular ventricular rhythm. In the elderly the significance of Wenckebach periods is much the same as for first degree AV block (see above).

57

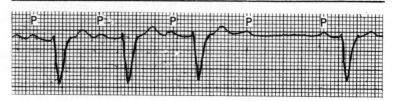

The Wenckebach phenomenon, 4:3 block – after the 4th P wave the QRS complex is lost

Figure 3.15

Mobitz type II block

In this much more unusual form of second degree heart block the heart remains in sinus rhythm and there are sporadic absences of the QRS complex following normal P waves. The P–R interval is fixed.

Significance   This form of heart block is of serious significance and is most commonly seen after acute myocardial infarction. It may, however, occur in patients who have only syncopal attacks or giddiness and in these it may also be a premonitory sign of complete heart block (see below). Some physicians believe that Mobitz type II block occurring after acute myocardial infarction is an indication for prophylactic temporary cardiac pacing.

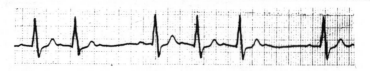

Mobitz type II block – fixed P–R interval (0.24 s) and intermittent absence of the QRS complex

Figure 3.16

High grade AV block (2:1, 3:1 heart block)

These types of second degree heart block fall outside Mobitz's original classification. There is normal sinus rhythm but only every other P wave (2:1 block) or every third P wave (3:1 block) is followed by a QRS complex.

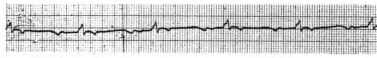

2:1 AV block

Figure 3.17

High grade AV block indicates serious disease of the conducting system. It may well be a premonitory sign of complete heart block, but may itself cause symptoms due to bradycardia. Occasionally it may be symptomless, especially in patients with digitalis intoxication. If symptoms occur the correct treatment is by insertion of a permanent cardiac pacemaker.

Treatment

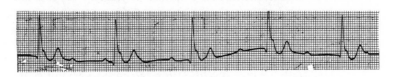

Complete heart block with idiojunctional rhythm

Figure 3.18

Third degree (complete) heart block

There is complete dissociation between the atrial and ventricular activity. Thus the P–R intervals constantly vary and the heart action is continued by means of an escape rhythm due to a focus of activity either in or, more usually, below the AV node. Thus there is usually an idioventricular escape rhythm and the QRS complexes show a right or left bundle branch block pattern.

Treatment

Complete heart block nearly always causes symptoms in the elderly, such as severe giddiness and syncopal attacks – the classical 'Stokes–Adams attacks'. In a very few patients there may be apparently no symptoms, but these are people who lead a totally sedentary life. Drug treatment with long-acting preparations of isoprenaline is unsatisfactory and the correct management is by insertion of a permanent cardiac pacemaker.

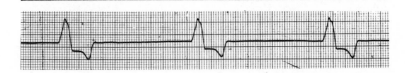

Idioventricular rhythm with no atrial activity

Figure 3.19

Bundle branch block

Interference with the conduction through the bundle of His, bundle branch block, is a common finding in the elderly. It is due to heart disease and cannot be regarded as a normal finding. Most frequently the cause is ischaemic heart disease, especially in left bundle branch block. However, bundle branch abnormalities may be due to primary myocardial disease such as Lenegre's syndrome, cardiomyopathy and senile cardiac amyloidosis. Right bundle branch block may also be due to an atrial septal defect, which may rarely still be seen in old age. The importance of recognizing bundle branch disease lies not only in the identification of the underlying pathology, but also as a possible precursor of more extensive conduction abnormalities such as trifascicular block.

Block of one of the main bundles of His is associated with specific abnormalities of the ventricular complex of the e.c.g. without disturbance of the heart rate and the P–R interval. The main features are widening of the QRS complexes to 0.12 s or more, distortion of the QRS complexes and ST segment depression and T wave inversion over the blocked ventricle.

Right bundle branch block

The QRS complexes are widened and in lead V1 there is an M-shaped complex due to slurring of the R wave into an RSR′ pattern as a result of delayed right ventricular conduction. In

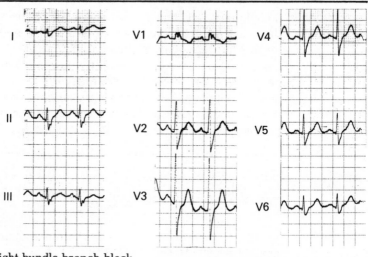

Figure 3.20 Right bundle branch block

the lateral chest leads, V5 and V6, and in leads I and aVL there is widening of the S wave. The T wave is inverted in lead V1. There is also generally deviation of the electrical axis to the right, where the deflection is usually negative in lead I and positive in leads II and III.

Left bundle branch block

The QRS complexes are widened in all leads and there are broad slurred R waves in leads I, aVL, V5 and V6. The S wave in leads V1 and V2 is deep and slurred. The T wave is inverted over the blocked left ventricle (V5 and V6). The ST segment take-off is elevated in leads V1 and V2.

The ST segment and T wave changes in LBBB are such that the uninitiated may mistake this for acute myocardial infarction, although of course, LBBB may be a result of this. The

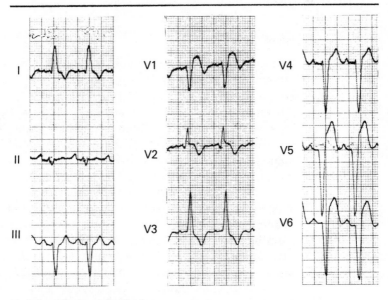

Left bundle branch block

Figure 3.21

cardinal feature of this condition is the widening of the QRS complexes and, as always, it is essential to examine each part of the e.c.g. cycle individually.

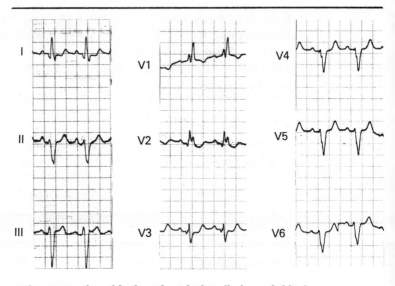

Figure 3.22 Left anterior hemiblock with right bundle branch block

Hemiblock

It has already been pointed out that the left bundle of His is a bifascicular branch and not infrequently only one fascicle may be blocked – usually the left anterior branch. This is known as left anterior hemiblock and may be recognized by extreme left axis deviation of greater than minus 30°. These changes imply a predominantly negative deflection in leads II and III. Sometimes left ventricular hypertrophy may produce a similar pattern. The importance of recognizing left anterior hemiblock is that it indicates serious conduction tissue disease and it is especially important when it is associated with right bundle branch block. When there is some conduction block of both main bundles, there is a risk of extension of this to involve the remainder of the His bundles, which will result in trifascicular block and a very slow ventricular rate. This is especially dangerous when there has been acute myocardial infarction and many authorities would regard this as an indication for prophylactic temporary cardiac pacing.

Cardiac pacemakers

The introduction of both temporary and permanent transvenous cardiac pacing has revolutionized the management of conduction disease in the heart and this is especially relevant in the elderly. The implantation rate of pacemakers varies considerably in different countries. The highest rate is in the United States and one of the lowest amongst the developed countries is in the United Kingdom. Since the rate of pacemaker implantation appears to be independent of the cost of health care, it can only be assumed that reasons for the variation is the failure to recognize the correct indications for pacing elderly patients in some countries. The techniques of cardiac pacing are beyond the scope of this book and similarly the different pacing generators that are available need no description. It is, however, necessary for the family doctor to understand something of the indications for pacing and also to be able to recognize some of the problems that may arise with artificial pacemakers.

Temporary cardiac pacing

Generally temporary pacing is only necessary in patients who have serious conduction disturbances that follow myocardial infarction and these are outlined in Chapter 2. The vast majority of conduction disturbances following myocardial infarction settle spontaneously after a week or so and only rarely do they persist and require permanent artificial pacing. Conduction disturbances occur most frequently after inferior wall infarction when there may be ischaemic changes in the atrioventricular node. Complete heart block is an absolute indication for temporary pacing after infarction and frequently high grade AV block (2:1, 3:1) leads to bradycardia and should be treated with a temporary pacemaker, whether there are symptoms of confusion, cerebral ischaemia or not, since the bradycardia results in decreased coronary artery perfusion and probably extension of the area of muscle damage. Many authors consider that the finding of Mobitz type II block after infarction is an indication for prophylactic temporary pacing, since unless treated many of these patients progress to complete heart block. Similarly the combination of right bundle branch block and left anterior hemiblock is a potentially dangerous situation, since if the only remaining fascicle of the left bundle is then involved, a very slow idioventricular rhythm supervenes and it is wise to consider these patients for temporary pacing.

The techniques of temporary cardiac pacing through the right subclavian vein are relatively simple and facilities for this should be available in every general hospital. Some physicians make a practice of inserting a temporary pacing electrode in patients at the local hospital before referring them to a cardiac centre for permanent pacing and this relieves the major centre of some emergency action and ensures that the patient with Stokes–Adams attacks has immediate protection before transfer.

Permanent cardiac pacing

Permanent cardiac pacing is used for patients with progressive degenerative changes in the conducting system. The technique is relatively simple and should be carried out in a cardiac centre. Permanent pacemakers are not cheap and involve continued follow-up and the indications for their implantation must be clear. Patients must understand the implications and limitations of this treatment as well as the great advantages that should accrue from it.

Indications for permanent pacing

The classical Stokes–Adams attack due to complete heart block is well-recognized as a major indication for pacing, but there are a few patients who have complete heart block without any symptoms of dizziness or faints and it is felt that truly asymptomatic patients should not be treated in this way, although they do need careful supervision. Any bradycardia due to AV nodal block with symptoms of dizziness, fits, faints or falls is a clear indication for pacing and these patients should be referred to the hospital. Many of these patients may have intermittent AV block, at least in the early stages of their symptoms, and the difficulties of diagnosis are discussed in Chapter 6.

   In recent years our understanding of the 'sick sinus syndrome' has advanced considerably and this is discussed in more detail above. Sinus node disease is increasingly common as age advances and may not be related to coronary artery disease. If sino-atrial block and the bradycardia–tachycardia syndrome give rise to symptoms then the most effective treatment is by implantation of a permanent pacemaker. In the case of the bradycardia–tachycardia syndrome it may also be necessary to give anti-arrhythmic drugs as well, although one must be a little careful since these agents may interfere with the pacemaker threshold.

The results of permanent cardiac pacing are extremely satisfactory and should result in complete alleviation of the patients' symptoms. The majority of pacemaker generators are of the 'on-demand' type which only operate when the patient's heart rate falls below a critical level. In the past many elderly patients were fitted with mercury cell batteries, which had a mean life of about two years. The usual practice nowadays is to fit lithium iodide powered generators, which should have a life expectancy of at least five years. The vast majority of units are inserted through the great veins into the right ventricle and the generator placed in the chest wall. In certain patients pacemaker electrodes are sutured directly on to the epicardium by open operation.

Pacemaker follow-up

In the past it has been customary for pacemaker generators to be assessed at a cardiac centre, but recently some local hospitals have been able to offer this service and in some cases it is possible to check the generators in the patient's home, with considerable saving of money and increased convenience to the patient. Pacemaker assessment locally is more effective since it is easier for the patients to attend local hospitals easily and frequently. The generators should be checked regularly one month, three months and then six monthly after leaving the cardiac centre. When the generator is approaching the end of its expected life, at 2, 5 or 8 years, it should be checked monthly. Performance checks are fairly simple and involve a simple e.c.g. rhythm strip and assessment by a battery analyser.

Complications of permanent pacemakers

The early complications of this treatment are few and usually only involve infection on the chest wall at the generator implantation site and more rarely slippage of the generator or skin necrosis, the latter which usually only occurs in very thin individuals. It is rare for the pacemaker electrode to become displaced from the right ventricular wall after the patient has left hospital.

Later complications are rare and are usually related to early failure of the generator. This should be detected by routine follow-up checks, but occasionally will occur suddenly. It is essential to remember that if any of the patient's original

symptoms recur then it is almost certainly due to pacemaker
failure and the patients should be carefully warned about this

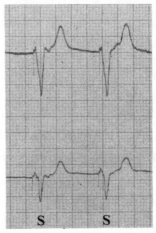

Figure 3.23 Artificial cardiac pacemaker: pacemaker spikes (P)

possibility. Suspected pacemaker failure should be treated as
an emergency and the patient referred immediately to hospital.
Most pacemakers tend to accelerate when the battery begins
to fail, although this is rarely detectable by simple pulse rate or
e.c.g. rhythm strip counting unless it is very advanced.

Sometimes after implantation there may be a rise in the
pacemaker threshold resulting in failure of the pacing spikes to
activate the ventricle ('missing'). This can be diagnosed from
the e.c.g. which shows a pacemaker spike which is not followed
by a QRST complex.

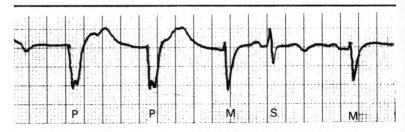

Pacemaker missing. Paced beats (P) followed by a missed pacemaker
beat (M) followed by a sinus beat (S)

Figure 3.24

Disorders of the cardiovascular system (III)

DISEASES OF THE ARTERIES

Coronary arteries: angina pectoris – Mesenteric artery insufficiency (mesenteric angina) – Diseases of the aorta – Peripheral vascular disease – Diabetic arterial disease – Giant cell arteritis (temporal arteritis)

Coronary arteries: angina pectoris

Although ischaemic heart disease is very common in the elderly, occurring in about 20% of men and 12% of women over the age of 65 years, the problem of angina appears to become progressively less as age advances. The reason for this phenomenon is probably largely explained by the fact that with increasing age exercise decreases and ischaemic heart pain is less readily induced. However, many elderly people do expect to take regular exercise and many continue to work. In these patients angina can seriously limit their activities and impair their quality of life. The investigation and management of angina is not significantly different in the elderly from the middle-aged patient.

Symptoms　　Angina is characterized by retrosternal pain on exertion that is relieved by rest. Rarely this pain may be atypical and may only occur in the lower jaw, shoulders or even the arms. Cardiac pain is discussed in more detail in the previous chapter and it is important to differentiate between this and other causes of chest pain.

Investigation　　Investigation of the patient with angina includes a thorough physical examination with special attention being paid to the presence of obesity, hypertension, valvular disease of the heart, diabetes and lipid abnormalities. A resting elec-

67

trocardiogram is mandatory and if normal, should be carefully repeated on exercise.

Treatment

Treatment of angina includes rectification, if possible, of the abnormalities listed above and general advice about activities and lifestyle. The proper use of sublingual trinitrin is essential; it must always be carried by the patient and used at the first indication of pain. If possible the prophylactic use of trinitrin when it is known that any particular exercise produces chest pain is very helpful. These simple remedies have

TNT been stressed because it is surprising how often patients with angina, seen in hospital, have never been properly advised about the use of this drug, or, if they have, appear to have forgotten the advice. There are long-acting forms of trinitrin available for prophylactic use and these may be helpful.

Sorbitrate It has only recently been realized that the potency of trinitrin deteriorates quite rapidly and if these tablets have been stored for more than a month or two they may be inactive. If the patient gets no associated headache or flushing when these tablets are sucked this may be a pointer to lack of potency. Thus it may be better to use chewable isosorbide dinitrate (Sorbitrate) tablets, which are effective in relieving angina. This preparation may also be taken prophylactically by swallowing one tablet four times a day.

β-blockers The introduction of the β-blocking agents in the 1960s has produced a real advance in the treatment of this condition and unless there are serious contraindications, such as obstructive airways disease, these drugs should be the first treatment aimed at reducing or abolishing the attacks. There is no convincing evidence that the dosage of these drugs in the elderly should be any different to that in younger people. A drug such as propranolol may be started in a dose of 10 mg three times a day and increased until the attacks are controlled. There may be some advantage of using long-acting preparations in the elderly to simplify treatment.

Nifedipine If β-blockers fail to control the anginal attacks it is worthwhile exhibiting nifedipine starting with a dose of 10 mg three times daily and doubling this if it is not completely effective. This drug can be given with β-blocking agents and may potentiate their effect. It is also useful to start with this drug if β-blockers are contraindicated.

One of the problems in patients with angina is that the

e.c.g. tracing may be normal, even on exercise, and the finding of a normal e.c.g. in no way excludes the diagnosis. This is especially relevant in 'crescendo' angina, when the attacks occur with increasing frequency and also occur at rest. There may be a case for anticoagulating these patients if they do not respond to bed rest and adequate β-blockade. Unless the home circumstances are good it may well be advisable to admit these patients to hospital for more intensive management.

Anti-
coagulants

With careful management patients with angina may be able to lead normal or nearly normal lives and longevity may not be seriously compromised. The coexistence of other diseases, such as diabetes mellitus adversely affects the prognosis and it is important to make sure that this is well controlled.

Mesenteric artery insufficiency (mesenteric angina)

Occlusive disease of the superior mesenteric artery is an important problem in the elderly and the diagnosis is frequently overlooked. It is included in this chapter because of its similarity, both pathologically and functionally, to coronary artery disease. Acute occlusion of the artery is usually fatal, but it is possible to recognize the subacute ischaemic episodes that occur with this disease and surgical operation at this stage is extremely satisfactory.

Symptoms

The symptoms of mesenteric artery insufficiency are most commonly of abdominal pain, the distribution of which is related to the segment of small or large bowel which is affected. This pain may be quite diffuse and is often colicky in nature. It is usually related to meals and sometimes to exercise. There is usually anorexia and weight loss and occasionally gastrointestinal bleeding and anaemia. There may be significant malabsorption in chronic cases. The bowel habit is frequently disturbed, either by constipation or diarrhoea. Clinical examination may be less helpful than the history, but the patient usually looks ill and thin, there is frequently anaemia and impaired peripheral pulses. Occasionally one may hear an abdominal aortic bruit.

Investigation

Investigation of mesenteric angina is difficult. There may be evidence of malabsorption and the barium meal may show disordered motility with puddling of barium. If the diagnosis is suspected then an aortogram will demonstrate the ischaemic lesions.

69

Treatment

The treatment of mesenteric artery insufficiency is surgical, usually by endarterectomy or bypass grafting. This may be urgent if the blood supply is so precarious that the slightest further impairment will precipitate extensive gangrene. If the acute situation occurs the outlook is extremely poor since patients do not tolerate extensive bowel gangrene for many hours and the widespread bowel resection that is necessary is often fatal anyway.

Diseases of the aorta

The vast majority of aortic disease is a result of degenerative and arteriosclerotic changes, but occasionally one still sees aortic disease as a result of tertiary syphilitic infection.

The thoracic aorta

Dilatation and aneurism of the ascending aorta are often caused by syphilitic disease and the clue is provided by the finding of calcification in the wall on chest X-ray. Arch aneurisms are more common and are the result of arteriosclerosis. The symptoms are usually those of pressure effects, either on the left innominate vein, causing unilateral elevation of the left jugular venous pulse, or involvement of the left recurrent laryngeal nerve causing hoarseness of the voice. Involvement of the hilar lymph glands by such diseases as carcinoma of the bronchus are very much more frequent causes of these symptoms, however. Aneurism of the descending thoracic aorta is a much less frequent site and this may cause dysphagia due to extrinsic pressure of the oesophagus just above the diaphragm.

Investigation   Investigation of disease of the thoracic aorta is by simple chest X-ray, and usually other diseases can be excluded by this or by tomography. A barium swallow conveniently outlines the oesophagus and excludes neoplasms of the oesophagus and achylasia of the cardia. With ascending thoracic aneurisms blood serology for syphilis must be checked.

Treatment

The management of these conditions poses great problems in elderly patients, since surgical correction is a major, and

70

usually unjustifiable, procedure. Tertiary syphilis should be treated with a full three week course of intramuscular penicillin. Dysphagia may be greatly helped by regular oesophageal dilatation.

Dissecting aneurism of the thoracic aorta has already been described in Chapter 2 and this accounts for about half the cases of aneurism of the ascending aorta.

The abdominal aorta

The abdominal aorta is frequently the site of considerable arteriosclerotic change and occasionally may be aneurismally dilated. Many of these patients have no symptoms referable to their disease. Occasionally the origin of the renal arteries are involved with signs of renal insufficiency. Much more frequently the distal abdominal aorta and the origins of the iliac arteries are the seat of atherosclerotic occlusive disease and this probably accounts for about a quarter of patients with intermittent claudication. Rarely the claudication is limited to the gluteal muscles and thighs with associated impotence (Leriche's syndrome). Clinically the femoral and distal pulses are reduced or even absent and there may be a bruit heard in the groins. The diagnosis can be confirmed by aortography and, if the symptoms are severe, surgical correction by means of bypass grafting is indicated, since there is no effective method of conservative management.

Peripheral vascular disease

This is a common and important condition in the elderly. The two main clinical problems are intermittent claudication and gangrenous changes. About two thirds of patients with peripheral vascular disease have occlusion of the femoral or popliteal arteries and about a quarter have occlusion of aorto-iliac system.

Symptoms   Generally the presenting symptom is of intermittent claudication, but occasionally it may be rest pain, which is usually burning and occurs at night. Rarely, gangrenous changes in the toes or in the heels in bedridden patients may be the first signs of peripheral vascular disease. The changes are progressive.

Clinical signs   The clinical signs are of pallor of the foot, loss of hair and atrophy of the nails. The peripheries are cold and often discoloured. Careful examination of the peripheral pulses is mandatory and may give some clue to the level of arterial occlusion. The presence of a bruit over the femoral artery or the abdominal aorta may indicate proximal disease. In some cases it may be possible to demonstrate areas of anaesthesia or muscle wasting. It is important to detail the degree of exercise intolerance.

Investigation   Investigation of peripheral vascular disease must include a general physical examination, including an e.c.g., since about a quarter of patients with intermittent claudication also have angina. All patients should have a chest X-ray, full blood count and ESR, blood sugar and blood urea estimations. All these investigations can be performed by the family doctor. If there is any question of surgical treatment by bypass grafting then the patient should be referred to a hospital for aortography. Thermography and radionuclide angiography may also have a place in investigation if they are available locally.

Differential diagnosis of peripheral vascular disease

In the elderly there are several conditions which may also produce limb pain and these include peripheral neuritis and lumbo-sacral nerve root irritation, usually from disc prolapse or the cauda equina syndrome. Osteoarthritis of the hip or knee and myxoedema may also mimic the symptoms of peripheral vascular disease and should be excluded. None of these conditions interferes with the peripheral pulses. Diabetic vasculitis should be excluded and this is discussed below.

Management of peripheral vascular disease

Medical   The natural history of chronic lower limb ischaemia is not nearly as serious as was believed in the past. In several large surveys medical management results in some improvement, even up to three years from the onset of symptoms and only about 10% of patients require some form of amputation in the first five years after presentation. Thus, in the elderly, conservative treatment is usually satisfactory.

The most important first step is to stop the patient smoking, as continued cigarette consumption is the single most likely factor to lead to the necessity for amputation. Local care of the feet is important, as any infection is likely to lead to serious complications. The services of a chiropodist are helpful in paring nails and treating corns. Treatment of polycythaemia and anaemia improve peripheral circulation, and weight reduction in obese patients is helpful. The use of vasodilator drugs is not usually indicated and indeed may worsen the situation by diverting blood flow to less ischaemic areas. Defibrinating and platelet anti-aggregating agents may be of some use. If there is evidence of embolism, as in patients with chronic or intermittent atrial fibrillation, anticoagulant drugs are indicated. It is essential to avoid the use of β-blocking agents, as these drugs may precipitate intermittent claudication. Recently there has been some evidence that cholesterol-lowering drugs such as clofibrate (Atromid) may be helpful in these patients and certainly the treatment of myxoedema, which results in a raised serum cholesterol level, will improve peripheral vascular insufficiency.

The great majority of elderly patients will continue to lead a satisfactory life with these measures, but in some people surgical intervention will be necessary. This may be corrective, such as lumbar sympathectomy or bypass grafting, or ablative, involving amputation.

Indications for surgery

Symptoms and signs of advanced ischaemia, such as severe rest pain or early gangrenous changes and rapidly progressive disease are indications for surgery. In this situation the family physician should immediately refer the patient to hospital. Even in the elderly there is a place for reconstructive surgery if the disease is localized, but this cannot be accurately identified without aortography. Even with generalized disease, lumbar sympathectomy may improve the condition for some months and allow a return to normal or near-normal life.

Embolism

If the disease is localized, thromboendarterectomy or bypass grafting is very satisfactory and age alone is no barrier to this sort of procedure. Arterial embolism may occur suddenly in an elderly person and is usually a sequel to recent myocardial infarction due to dislodging of a mural thrombus, or a result of chronic or intermittent atrial fibrillation. If the patient is fit enough emergency embolectomy is indicated and the decision to refer the patient to hospital must be made immediately. These patients should also be put on longterm anticoagulant treatment.

Amputation

Amputation of part of a limb is an irreversible procedure and the decision as to when to operate and how extensive this

73

should be must be the decision of the surgeon, but the family physician has a part to play in this decision, since he will know the social and domestic background of the patient. Whilst too limited amputation may lead to further and often fatal ablation if gangrene recurs, the site of amputation may have very significant consequences for the patient. For example, a very old and frail patient may never regain independence following an above-knee amputation, but might well do so if it is possible to limit the surgery to below the knee with a long posterior flap procedure.

Rehabilitation
It is important for the patient about to undergo amputation to fully understand how independent it is now possible to become with modern protheses and proper rehabilitation techniques. Since amputation is nearly always an elective procedure there should be plenty of time to acquaint the patient with all the advantages and the very few disadvantages of the operation. It is always very worthwhile arranging an interview with an amputee who has been successfully rehabilitated, as many of the fears of the operation can be alleviated. Although there are some very elderly patients who have managed to learn to walk again despite bilateral above-knee amputation, this is exceptional, but most patients, however old, should be able to walk again after below- or through-knee amputation. Even if this is not possible it is important for the patient to know that with modern gadgetry an independent wheelchair existence is perfectly possible at home. The family physician's unique knowledge of the patient's background is extremely useful in these circumstances.

Amputation is mandatory where there is extensive and irreversible gangrene and bearing in mind the above observations, it is an operation which must be timed carefully and before the patient has deteriorated to a point where there is little hope of recovery and rehabilitation.

Diabetic arterial disease

There is a close relationship between diabetes and arterial disease and about 20% of patients with peripheral vascular disease have diabetes. The outlook for patients with diabetes and peripheral arterial insufficiency is infinitely worse than in those patients who have no disturbance of sugar metabolism. The reasons for this phenomenon are multiple and are primarily due to the development of peripheral neuropathy, infection and accelerated atherosclerosis. Thus there is a great need to maintain very careful control of the blood sugar.

Clinical features
The clinical features of diabetic peripheral vascular disease are different in several important ways from those patients without diabetes. Many diabetic patients have neuropathic or infected gangrene with relatively good circulation down to the level of demarcation. The peripheral pulses may often remain palpable and it is the microcirculation that is involved. However, diabetics may simply have the same picture as the senile arteriosclerotic patient.

Management
The management of these diabetics is different from the senile arteriosclerotic patients. It is advisable to treat them in hospital, since control of the local infection, bed rest and rigid control of blood sugar levels, often with insulin, are difficult to manage at home.

Prognosis
The prognosis for the ischaemic limb in diabetics is poor and the amputation rate is two to three times higher than for non-diabetics. The outlook for the other leg is also bad and as many as a quarter of the patients have to have a bilateral amputation within a year or two. Thus there is a need to rehabilitate these patients after amputation as quickly as possible so that they can enjoy a reasonable quality of life at home for the longest possible time. Physiotherapy aimed at strengthening the good leg before operation, together with immediate walking exercises using a temporary early walking aid after the operation will go a long way to achieving this goal.

Giant cell arteritis (temporal arteritis)

This is an important and common disease in the elderly, and is a good example of a condition that can be diagnosed and treated very satisfactorily out of hospital.

There is some evidence that giant cell arteritis is related to polymyalgia rheumatica (see Chapter 7) and certainly some patients present with all the symptoms of both diseases. The disease is virtually confined to the elderly and is much more common in women than in men. It is a disease that affects many systems and is characterized by giant cell infiltration of the media and intima of small arteries.

Symptoms
The disease generally presents with headache and sometimes visual disturbances, such as transient loss or blurring of vision. Many patients complain of tenderness of the scalp, which is commonly precipitated by combing the hair.

75

Patients are usually generally unwell, sometimes with fever, anorexia and weight loss. The girdle pain and stiffness of polymyalgia rheumatica may also be present.

Examination   Clinical examination shows the presence of tenderness over the temporal artery, which may be thickened. If the disease is not rapidly diagnosed and treated there may be evidence of central retinal artery occlusion. The ESR is almost always raised, usually in the range of 60–90 mm in the first hour. Biopsy of the temporal artery generally confirms the diagnosis, but if the disease is strongly suspected, treatment should not be withheld to await the pathology report, or indeed stopped even if it is negative.

Treatment

Treatment should immediately be started with corticosteroids, using a drug such as prednisolone orally in a starting dose of 60 mg per day in divided doses. Practically all patients should get immediate relief of their symptoms within 48 hours, and the ESR falls rapidly. The dose of prednisolone can be reduced quite quickly once the disease is controlled, but it is necessary to continue treatment with a maintenance dose of 5 – 10 mg for at least a year and probably for much longer since relapses are not uncommon after cessation of therapy.

5 Strokes

*Predisposing factors to stroke – Pathophysiology of stroke –
Transient ischaemic attacks (TIAs) – The stroke in evolution –
The completed stroke*

Cerebrovascular disease is a major cause of mortality and morbidity throughout the world and is exceeded only by ischaemic heart disease and cancer as a cause of death in developed countries. It is not so much the immediate mortality, but the continued survival of patients with strokes that will concern the family physician to a greater degree. An acute stroke is a catastrophe for both the patient and his relatives and survival from the stroke may present a major burden on medical resources. Family physicians should be familiar with the management of cerebrovascular disease because a positive approach will yield great benefit to the patient.

Early diagnosis of the incomplete stroke may enable treatment to arrest further evolution of the disease and recognition of transient ischaemic attacks can usually lead to the abolition of further attacks with correct treatment. Management of the completed stroke will require a great deal of skill and the co-ordination of rehabilitation and social services in order to assist maximum recovery of function and to deal with any residual disability. Accumulating knowledge in the last few years suggests that there is much more that we can now do to modify not only the incidence and disability of stroke disease, but to improve the lifestyle of those patients who do have residual functional loss.

Incidence   Cerebrovascular accidents may occur at any age, but the

77

incidence rises exponentially with age, being slightly higher in men than in women. In the United Kingdom the incidence of stroke is about three per 1000 in the 55–64 year age group, eight per 1000 in those aged between 65 and 74 and 25 per 1000 in those aged 75 years and over. This pattern is seen in most Western countries, although there are both racial and regional variations. For example, in the USA stroke rates are higher in blacks than in whites and there are consistently higher rates in the south-eastern states from Maine to Georgia. This regional variation is also seen in the United Kingdom, where the incidence of stroke is higher in the north than in the south.

Mortality

After the age of 60 years the incidence of stroke becomes the same as that of ischaemic heart disease and after the age of 70 years it is more common. The mortality rate for strokes has been falling in the Western world for some time and the reason for this is not clearly understood, but it has resulted in an increase in the number of people affected by stroke disease surviving in the community. In a standard population one would expect up to two new strokes per 1000 people per year and there will be about another five patients who will have had a stroke sometime in the past and who have survived. Since the incidence of stroke is much higher in those over 65 years than in younger age groups, a family physician with a higher than average proportion of patients over this age will expect to have to deal with relatively more people with this problem.

Predisposing factors to stroke

The possible causative factors in stroke disease have been the subject of much research, but, although some positive findings have emerged in young and middle-aged persons, in the elderly, in whom strokes are most frequent, the evidence for definite causal factors is conflicting.

TIAs

The occurrence of a previous stroke or transient ischaemic attack makes the likelihood of a further episode much more common and it is, therefore, essential to investigate and treat transient ischaemic attacks. There is little doubt that hypertension in people below the age of 60 years is associated with an increased incidence of stroke, especially in men. Thus therapeutic control of the blood pressure in this group is indicated. However, the benefit of blood pressure control in women is less clear, and in those aged 65 years and over there is at present little evidence that the level of blood pressure is

Blood
pressure

related to the incidence of strokes. There is currently a large prospective study of the European Working Party on Hypertension taking place which may give a clearer answer to this problem.

Smoking

There is little doubt that smoking in younger men is associated with a higher than average incidence of stroke, but in the elderly this association is not clear. Because of the fire hazard of smoking in the elderly and the risk of respiratory disease, it is probably worth stopping the older patient from smoking on general grounds anyway. Smoking also raises the

Haematocrit

haematocrit, and this is a recognized risk factor for stroke. It is certain that high levels of haemoglobin and packed cell volume should be treated by venesection (see Chapter 12).

Diabetes

The coexistence of diabetes mellitus that requires treatment is associated with an increased incidence of stroke. There is, however, no evidence to suggest that minor degrees of glucose intolerance are related to vascular disturbances and from this point of view their detection is irrelevant.

Obesity

Obesity and high levels of blood lipids do not appear to be related to the incidence of stroke. It is wise to treat obesity, however, on general grounds, and especially in those who have had a stroke since it will improve the functional recovery.

Water hardness

There is some evidence from Japan and some Western countries that water hardness has some protective action against both ischaemic heart disease and stroke, but the mechanism of this association remains an area of considerable conjecture.

Pathophysiology of stroke

Cerebral blood flow

Strokes are caused by local interference of cerebral blood flow. The degree of cerebral necrosis will to some extent depend on the degree of collateral circulation that is available to the

Collateral circulation

affected area through the circle of Willis. Even occlusion of major arterial branches may result in little neurological impairment if the collateral circulation is good. Strokes usually occur when there is widespread arterial disease, whether extracranial or intracranial. There is some 'autoregulation' of

Auto-regulation

cerebral blood flow achieved by the constriction or dilatation of cerebral arterioles. This is related to systemic arterial pressure. At very low systemic pressures, when cerebral arteriolar dilatation is maximal, any further fall of blood pressure will reduce cerebral blood flow. In patients with raised arterial pressure the autoregulatory mechanism may be set at a higher level and in these people attempts to lower the systemic blood pressure may result in a reduction of cerebral blood flow which would not occur in a normal subject at the same pressure. The autoregulatory mechanism functions far less efficiently in the elderly as a result of degenerative changes in the cerebral arterial tree.

Strokes are often the result of occlusion of the carotid or vertebrobasilar arterial trees. The territories of these systems are separate and are connected only by the circle of Willis. More widespread neurological lesions are produced by embolic phenomena. Occlusion of the internal carotid artery results in hemiplegia affecting both upper and lower limbs, often with some sensory loss and is indistinguishable from occlusion of the middle cerebral artery. If the lesion affects the dominant hemisphere there will be interference with speech and often hemianopia. Occlusion of the anterior cerebral branch of the internal carotid artery usually affects the leg more severely than the arm. There may also be frontal lobe signs, such as sphincter involvement with incontinence and a positive grasp reflex. Transient attacks of blindness in one eye (amaurosis fugax) indicate that the internal carotid artery is affected since the opthalmic artery is one of its branches.

The vertebrobasilar system supplies the brain stem and occlusion of this artery give rise to vertigo, diplopia, facial parasthesiae, ataxia and dysarthria. There may be bilateral motor impairment in the limbs either with or without sensory loss. Hemianopia may also result as the posterior cerebral artery supplies the visual cortex.

Strokes may be a result of vascular disease caused by atheromatous plaques in the main arteries, especially the aorta, carotid and vertebrobasilar arteries, as well as the anterior and middle cerebral arteries. These plaques may either produce thrombus formation, or ulcerate and give rise to emboli, which then become lodged in smaller vessels.

Hypertension produces atheromatous plaques in the main arteries, but also affects the smaller arteries and arterioles. The weakness in the vessel wall produced by these changes may lead to the formation of small aneurisms and these may rupture and cause cerebral haemorrhage or block the vessels.

Emboli may arise from the major arteries in the neck affected by atheromatous changes, but also occur as a result of heart disease. In atrial fibrillation, especially when associated with mitral valve disease, thrombus formation may develop in the non-functioning atria. These may become dislodged and

Margin notes: Internal carotid artery · Vertebro-basilar artery · Atheroma · Hypertensive vascular disease · Emboli

embolize to the brain, especially if the atrial fibrillation is intermittent. Occasionally a mural thrombus may occur in the left ventricle following myocardial infarction. From time to time fragments of these mural thrombi may be thrown into the circulation and pass into the cerebral vessels.

A small proportion of strokes are caused by other pathology; the most important of which are the collagen diseases such as giant cell arteritis, cerebral tumours and subdural haematomata.

Transient ischaemic attacks (TIAs)

A TIA is a focal neurological disturbance lasting less than 24 hours. These lesions are nearly always recurrent and it is therefore important to recognize and treat them as soon as possible.

The neurological disturbance is of abrupt onset and may last only a few minutes. Recovery is usually rapid and complete. The TIA may arise as a result of disturbed blood flow in either the carotid or vertebrobasilar systems. The symptoms and physical signs are, therefore, localized in the same way as completed strokes due to occlusion of these vessels. In a TIA, however, the physical signs of upper motor neurone involvement are usually absent by the time that the patient sees the doctor, although there may be some lingering clue, such as an upgoing plantar response. The history is all-important.

Cardiac arrhythmia Hypotension

The other major causes of TIAs are transient cardiac arrhythmias and postural hypotension. Cardiac arrhythmias are often difficult to diagnose and are discussed in more detail in Chapter 3. The finding of a normal e.c.g. does not exclude them. Postural hypotension is usually a result of drug treatment. Cranial arteritis may also cause TIAs and it is essential to measure the ESR in all these patients.

Transient ischaemic attacks involving the carotid artery territory carry a worse prognosis than those of the vertebrobasilar system. A clear history is essential. Sometimes a bruit may be heard over the lesion in the carotid artery. Once the diagnosis is made treatment should be instituted. Further investigation in the elderly should be limited, since very few of these patients will be good candidates for carotid endarterectomy.

Treatment

Treatment of carotid TIAs involves the removal of the cause,

Carotid TIAs

Vertebro-
basilar TIAs

whether this is due to cranial arteritis, transient cardiac arrhythmias or postural hypotension. If this is not relevant, treatment can either be with anticoagulants, such as warfarin, or with a combination of aspirin and dipyridamole (Persantin).

Lesions affecting the vertebrobasilar territory are much less likely to proceed to completed strokes and the treatment can be less aggressive. In these circumstances aspirin and dipyridamole may be helpful, especially if there are long tract signs. Cardiac arrhythmias need to be excluded by prolonged ambulatory monitoring and a cervical collar may help those who have mechanical deformation of the vertebral arteries from cervical spondylosis. Labyrinthine sedatives are usually helpful, e.g. cinnarizine (Stugeron), in relieving the vertigo. Rarely the subclavian steal syndrome may cause a vertebrobasilar TIA, and can be suspected if exercise of the arm reproduces the symptoms. There may be inequality of the radial pulses and a bruit may be heard over the subclavian artery above the clavicle.

The stroke in evolution

Sometimes a stroke may develop slowly over several hours. In this situation it may be possible to modify the course of the disease by giving anticoagulant therapy. The presence of polycythaemia can be treated by emergency venesection. It is essential to exclude haemorrhage as the cause of the stroke in evolution and a lumbar puncture to examine the cerebrospinal fluid (CSF) should be performed. Occasionally a subdural haematoma or a cerebral tumour may present in this way. A subdural haematoma as a result of a previous head injury usually leads to some variability in conscious level and the drowsiness is out of proportion to the upper motor neurone signs. The history of head injury has usually been forgotten by the patient or passed unnoticed by friends and relatives. If anticoagulants are to be given one should start with intravenous heparin and follow this with warfarin, and this should be undertaken in hospital.

The completed stroke

The completed stroke is the commonest way in which the patient will present. The site of the lesion and the underlying pathology can usually be assessed satisfactorily at home by clinical and electrocardiographic examination. A measured high blood pressure after a completed stroke may not necessarily indicate established hypertension. Similarly, T wave inversion on the e.c.g. does not always imply that the patient has had a myocardial infarction, since a cerebrovascular accident may produce widespread T wave inversion.

Prognosis

Overall about 50% of patients with completed strokes will die in the first few weeks, but the majority of these are those who have had a cerebral haemorrhage. Since intensive investigation is not often indicated in the elderly for the reasons outlined above, admission to hospital is indicated largely on social grounds. It may be impossible to nurse a patient with a major stroke at home, since an unconscious or semiconscious patient will need to be nursed semi-prone to maintain an adequate airway and will need regular turning to prevent pressure sores. If unconsciousness persists for more than a day, fluid and nutriment will need to be given by naso-gastric tube, and this can only be done satisfactorily in a nursing home or hospital. Simple physiotherapy by passively moving the affected limbs to prevent contractures can be performed by the relatives or even the patient himself. Proper positioning of the limbs is also important to prevent the development of deformities. Thus in the severe stroke it is probably better to transfer the patient to hospital.

Indications for hospital admission

Drug treatment

There are no indications for specific drug treatment in the acute completed stroke. If an embolism has been shown to cause the stroke, anticoagulants should be started orally after three to four weeks, provided there are no contraindications. The use of cerebral vasodilators and dexamethasone are not indicated in this situation. The treatment of raised arterial blood pressure is the subject of debate, but if any drug is to be used a diuretic should first be given, as there is no indication to reduce the blood pressure rapidly, whatever its level.

Prognosis for recovery of function

Once the stroke and the patient's condition have become stabilized, active physiotherapy should be started as soon as possible, with the aim of restoring the fullest physical, mental and social capability possible. The greatest improvement that can be expected will occur in the first three months, but continued recovery may occur up to two years. At least half of the affected patients should make a good recovery and become independent. About a quarter of the patients should achieve a reasonable degree of independence, but will need some help. Less than one quarter will remain severely disabled.

Neglect of affected side

One of the major causes of slow rehabilitation is the patient's neglect of the affected side of the body. Sometimes this will be ascribed to a hemianopia, but this is often not the case.

Great efforts should be made to make the patient aware of his affected side and relatives should be encouraged to approach the patient from this side and as far as possible to remove sensory stimuli from the good side. Impairment of speech and intellect will also hinder recovery and expert speech therapy has an important part to play in rehabilitation.

Speech therapy

The maintenance of balance reflexes is important in all old people during immobilization and especially in stroke disease. At the earliest moment the patient should be sat out of bed and walking exercises begun. Walking aids are useful, especially a frame as it encourages use of the affected upper limb. Spasticity may be a problem and can often be helped by drugs, such as dantrilene (Dantrium) or diazepam (Valium). If possible, splinting should be avoided as this increases the spasm. For some unexplained reason the degree of improvement in the upper limb is usually much less than in the lower.

Exercises

Spasticity

Occupational therapy will play an important role in rehabilitation and like physiotherapy, can be available on either an out-patient or in-patient basis. If the social circumstances are satisfactory at home and the degree of stroke is not too severe, patients will probably progress at least as fast at home as in hospital. Referral to outpatient occupational therapy departments or a Day Hospital will enable the patient to regain morale, as well as progressing towards independence in his activities of daily living such as dressing, cooking and the maintenance of mobility and continence. It should also be possible for the patient to regain more complex industrial skills in the Day Hospital or occupational therapy department, if this is relevant. Much of the simpler work of physiotherapists and occupational therapists can be performed by the patient's relatives at home.

Rehabilitation

Thus the aim of treatment, to regain maximum independence, is a reality for most patients with stroke disease. If initial hospital admission is necessary, it should still be the aim for early discharge to home. The family physician is in a good position to help this. He will know the family and can counsel them; he will know the patient's home circumstances and will be able to ensure that adequate support from nurses and other bodies are available and that the necessary aids to support independent living are provided. Even with severe residual functional deficit only a few patients need to stay in hospital.

Summary

Cerebrovascular disease is a major cause of death and disability. Strokes are caused by local disturbances of blood flow as a result of haemorrhage, thrombosis or embolism. Two main patterns of neurological deficit occur; from occlusive disease of the carotid or vertebrobasilar artery territory. Strokes may be transient (TIAs) in evolution or completed. Investigation and treatment of carotid TIAs are urgent since they frequently progress to completed stroke. Embolism, cardiac arrhythmias, postural hypotension and cranial arteritis are amongst the more important treatable causes of TIAs.

The management of the completed stroke is discussed and the indications for admission to hospital, the place of drug treatment and the role of therapists and family outlined. The aid of treatment is the reinstatement of independent living and in the majority of patients this can be achieved.

Fits, faints and falls

Definitions – Fits – Faints – Falls

These are very common symptoms and constitute an important problem area for family physicians and specialist physicians alike. The evaluation of these symptoms and their treatment are often difficult, but with careful history-taking and examination many patients can be considerably improved and not infrequently cured. The first pitfall in diagnosis lies in the wide variation that patients, and sometimes doctors, have in the interpretation of the attacks. For example, one person may describe a 'faint' as a transient period of dizziness or light-headedness, but another may consider it to be a fall with a period of unconsciousness.

Definitions

It is important that the doctor and the patient understand that they are talking about the same thing and it may be helpful if the doctor explains the terminology to the patient. A 'fit' implies a period of altered consciousness and is due to sudden paroxysmal discharge from neurones. Epileptic fits may be either idiopathic or symptomatic of diseases such as cerebral tumours or cerebral arteriosclerosis. The presentation of a fit may be local, as in temporal lobe or Jacksonian epilepsy, or generalized, as in petit mal or grand mal seizures. Temporal lobe, or psychomotor fits, are characterized by subjective awareness of visual or auditory hallucinations or illusions associated with disorientation and confusion; there may also be memory disturbance such as the *déjà vu* phenomenon. There may be a degree of automatism and the patient may carry out

Fits

Temporal lobe

87

well co-ordinated and purposeful actions without having any subsequent memory of them.

Jacksonian   Jacksonian fits have a focal origin and the seizure slowly spreads to adjacent parts of the body according to their representation in the cerebral cortex. The spread may be self-limiting or progress into a generalized convulsion.

Petit mal   Petit mal attacks are unusual in the elderly and consist of a transitory impairment of consciousness or 'absence' during normal activity. They often pass unnoticed by both the patient and observer. There may be twitching of the eyelids or rolling of the eyeballs and occasionally a more prolonged period of automatism.

Grand mal   Grand mal fits are usually preceded by an aura followed by the tonic phase, where the patient becomes rigid and unconscious. The clonic phase rapidly follows and there are generalized jerking contractions. There is a period of cyanosis, frothing at the mouth, incontinence of urine and sometimes of faeces, and tongue biting. Occasionally the unconsciousness may last for some time and the patient is flaccid. Natural sleep may follow and on waking there is no recollection of the event. There may also be a period of post-epileptic automatism or strange behaviour.

Faints   A 'faint' or syncopal episode implies a transient loss of consciousness without the features of epilepsy. It is important to distinguish this from vertigo or dizziness. Fainting is due to a sudden reduction in cerebral blood flow and may be caused by a large number of disorders, the most important of which are both identifiable and treatable and are defined in the following paragraphs.

Vaso-vagal attacks   Vaso-vagal attacks are common and may be caused by strong emotional stimuli, such as the sight of blood or pain. Hot stuffy atmospheres may be frequent predisposing factors. There is a feeling of weakness and light-headedness and nausea. The patient is pale and clammy and the blood pressure is low. The loss of consciousness lasts a second or so. Other abnormal vagal responses that may occur are cough or micturition syncope.

Postural hypotension   Postural hypotension may also cause a faint and is due to many conditions, drug therapy, electrolyte disturbances and Addison's disease, varicose veins, blood loss and simply degenerative changes in the autonomic nervous system being the most important.

The most difficult causes of faints to diagnose are those involving extra-cranial artery insufficiency, including the

88

subclavian steal syndrome and transient cardiac arrhythmias. These are described in more detail below.

Falls   'Falls' imply a sudden deviation from the normal erect posture and may be caused by any of the above-mentioned conditions. Very often, however, they may be accidental due to tripping over hidden obstacles or slipping on loose mats on polished surfaces. They may be frequently associated with abnormal locomotor function and occur in patients with central nervous system disorders such as Parkinson's disease and stroke and in those with osteoarthritis, especially of the hip and knee joints.

Evaluation of the history

Patients often have great difficulty in describing these episodes accurately. There is a problem not only in remembering the exact sequence of events, but also in reporting the frequency and timing of the attacks. It is vital to interview friends and relatives, especially if they have witnessed one or more episodes. If the falls are frequent it is worth getting the patient

Falls diary   or an observer to keep a 'falls diary' and to chart the timing, any unusual features and accompanying symptoms of the attacks. A falls diary is certainly a useful method of assessing the effect of treatment and should be used in the same way as a diabetic patient charts his urine tests.

Fits

Idiopathic epilepsy is rare in the elderly and an underlying cause for fits must be sought. Petit mal attacks are uncommon and the family doctor will be concerned primarily with local or generalized fits. Major attacks will be seen occasionally as

Stroke   part of an acute stroke caused by cerebrovascular disease, but they are also an important presenting feature of cerebral

Tumours,   tumours. Unless there are other obvious causes for an epileptic
primary   fit full investigation is indicated. This includes a thorough neurological examination. A general physical examination is important to exclude primary malignant lesions elsewhere with secondary deposits in the brain – lesions commonly mis-

Secondary   sed are carcinomas of the lung and bowel. Providing that there are no signs of raised intracranial pressure a lumbar puncture should be performed. Skull radiographs may be useful, but the electroencephalogram rather less so. To some extent invasive investigations such as carotid arteriography have been replaced by non-invasive tests, of which computerized axial tomography (CAT) scans are the best known, but isotope scans, thermography and ultrasound techniques have an important, although less evaluated, place in investigation.

In recent years it has become apparent that many cases of late-onset epilepsy are caused by transient interference with cardiac output, usually as a result of arrhythmias and intermittent heart block. Very often these disturbances are difficult to identify from the history, clinical examination, and even on inspection of the resting 12 lead electrocardiogram. The wider availability of ambulatory 24 hour cardiac monitoring (d.c.g.) has clearly shown that transient cardiac rhythm disturbances may be an important cause of epilepsy in the elderly, and they may also account for many faints and falls. This technique is discussed in detail elsewhere (Chapter 3) and should be considered a fundamental part of the investigation of epilepsy.

Heart block
Arrhythmias

The treatment of fits

In the vast majority of older patients the treatment will be that of the underlying condition; for example there is no point in giving antiepileptic drugs to a patient who has transient heart block as a cause of the fits. Neurosurgery is indicated for those with primary resectable cerebral tumours. Even in patients with inoperable tumours a comfortable and worthwhile remission may be achieved with chemotherapy or corticosteroid treatment with either beta- or dexamethazone. For secondary malignant tumour deposits in the brain the outlook for the patient is usually very bleak, but there are some tumours, for example of the breast, when hormonal or chemotherapeutic agents may provide useful palliative treatment. In many instances aggressive therapy is not indicated and dexamethazone and anti-epileptic drugs may provide a welcome, albeit temporary, relief.

Epilepsy due to cerebrovascular disease can usually be well controlled by the administration of phenytoin (Epanutin) in a dose of 100–300 mg per day in divided doses. It is important to adjust the dosage by monitoring the blood levels of this drug, because although drowsiness is not often a problem with this agent, overdosage can cause serious ataxia. There is no indication to treat the first attack, as this may be an isolated phenomenon in cerebrovascular disease, but second and subsequent fits do require control by drugs. In the elderly

Phenytoin

90

Carbamaza-
pine
Primidone
Phenobarbi-
tone

phenytoin is the least toxic drug and is very effective in the correct dosage, but others that may be useful are carbamazapine (Tegretol), primidone (Mysoline) and phenobarbitone. There is no real advantage of giving combinations of these drugs in the great majority of patients. It is also worth mentioning that both phenytoin and primidone may cause a megaloblastic anaemia if used for prolonged periods. If a patient has been free of fits for five years it is perfectly reasonable to try to wean him slowly off treatment. No person with epilepsy should be allowed to drive a motor vehicle unless he has been free of attacks for at least three years.

Diazepam

Status epilepticus, or repeated fits, constitutes a medical emergency and is best treated with intravenous diazapam 10 mg. Thiopentone (Pentothal) is also effective, but should not be given unless an anaesthetist is available. Phenytoin may also be given intravenously if necessary.

Epilepsy due to transient cardiac arrhythmias is effectively treated by remedying the underlying cause and this subject is dealt with more fully in Chapter 3. There is no need to give anti-epileptic drugs in this situation.

Faints

Faints may be due to many causes and the most important are listed below. The investigation of these attacks can usually be conveniently carried out without admission to a hospital.

Extracranial artery disease

This syndrome is due to the narrowing of one or more of the extracranial arteries supplying the circle of Willis and is usually due to atheromatous change. The most common sites of obstruction are in the vertebral and common carotid arteries in the neck. This disease does not always result in fainting, but is conveniently dealt with in this section. The classical vertebrobasilar syndrome produces episodic symptoms and may involve function of the brain stem, occipital cortex or temporal lobe. Vertigo and ataxia are the most common symptoms, but there may be visual hallucinations, diplopia and visual field defects as well. Bulbar involvement causing dysphagia and dysphasia may occasionally occur and rarely there may be a transient hemiplegia. The sudden and transient 'drop attack'

Diagnosis

is an important feature of this syndrome. The diagnosis of this condition is made from the history and the symptoms and signs described above; very rarely there may be a vertebral artery bruit heard, but of more use is the precipitation of the symptoms by turning and extension of the neck.

Subclavian steal syndrome

The subclavian steal syndrome may mimic vertebrobasilar disease and is due to narrowing of the proximal part of the subclavian artery. This results in the shunting of blood retrogradely in the ipsilateral vertebral artery during exercise of the arm (see Figure 6.1), with consequent starvation of blood flow in the basilar artery. There may be unequal radial pulses and occasionally one may hear a subclavian bruit.

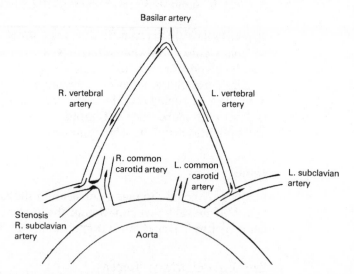

The subclavian steal syndrome showing reverse blood flow in right vertebral artery

Figure 6.1

Carotid artery stenosis

Carotid artery stenosis may also give rise to faints or 'transient ischaemic attacks' and is due to either atheromatous narrowing of the artery, most frequently at the origin of the common carotid tree, resulting in impaired blood flow, or it may be due to microemboli being thrown off from an atheromatous plaque on the endothelium. Apart from drop attacks, symptoms may vary from transient loss of vision on one side to frank episodes of hemiplegia with rapid recovery. The diagnosis is made from the history and there may be a bruit heard over the artery.

More exact definition of the arterial block may be made from aortic arch or carotid arteriography, but these procedures have some risk and should not be used unless there is some likelihood of performing arterial surgery. Newer, non-invasive investigations such as thermography and ultrasound will probably have an increasing place in the assessment of these arterial problems in the future.

The treatment of extracranial artery disease

Accurate diagnosis is essential and the avoidance of precipitating causes may result in considerable improvement. Vertebrobasilar disease is often helped by immobilizing the neck by means of a soft or plastazote collar. Plastazote is more effective, but many patients find these collars very uncomfortable and it is important to cover them with tubegauze which can be changed frequently. This method is often helpful as degenerative changes in the cervical spine may well exacerbate the condition by pinching the narrowed vertebral arteries. Subclavian steal disease and carotid artery stenosis are best treated by endarterectomy.

Aspirin

Considerable debate remains concerning the merits of drug manipulation of blood coagulability. There is some evidence that patients may be helped by alterations of platelet stickiness. Soluble aspirin 300 mg daily and dipyrimidole (Persantin) 100 mg three times daily or sulphinpyrazone (Anturan) 200 mg four times daily may well be tried without fear of significant side effects. In patients with more recurrent and

Anti-coagulants

severe symptoms of transient ischaemic attacks the use of anti-coagulants, such as warfarin or phenindione, may be indicated. The dangers of anticoagulants in the elderly have been greatly exaggerated in the past and age of itself has no relevance to the use of these drugs; obviously if there are other diseases present which may lead to dangerous bleeding, then they are contraindicated.

Venesection

In recent years venesection has tended to be used much less than formerly, but it is now increasingly recognized that hyperviscosity may be a real problem in patients with arterial insufficiency. If it is found that the haemoglobin value is greater than 18 g/100 ml and the haematocrit greater than 54% in patients with arterial insufficiency it is worth trying the effect of blood-letting.

Transient cardiac arrhythmias and conduction defects

Rhythm and conduction disturbances of the heart are important causes of fainting attacks and are considered in greater detail in Chapter 3. The classical Stokes–Adams attack due to complete heart block is usually easy to diagnose, but transient intermittent degrees of heart block are extremely difficult to demonstrate without ambulatory cardiac monitoring, because when the patient is examined the pulse rate is usually normal and the e.c.g. may show no abnormality. Similarly transient bradycardias and tachycardias or an alternating combination of both (the 'bradycardia–tachycardia' syndrome) are frequently missed by the most careful and expert examination and can only be demonstrated by 24-hour ambulatory monitoring. It is important to have a high index of suspicion in these patients, as many will admit to no history of palpitations. Ambulatory cardiac monitoring is an essential investigation in patients whose faints have no obvious cause.

Disorders of vagal response

Cough and micturition syncope are relatively uncommon and carotid hypersensitivity is rarely seen in practice. Cough syncope may be seen less often nowadays because chronic lung disease in the elderly is much less prevalent than formerly, but
Cough and micturition syncope
it still occurs and should be easily recognized as the faints are related to paroxysms of coughing. Micturition syncope most frequently occurs in men when they get up to urinate in the night. This fainting may well be related to postural hypotension (see below). Carotid sinus hypersensitivity, which usually occurs in men when they shave with concurrent extension of the neck, is probably more frequently caused by vertebrobasilar insufficiency. Carotid sinus massage, which should only be done with direct e.c.g. monitoring, will mimic the symptoms and a reflex sinus bradycardia will be demonstrated. This abnormal vagal response is a manifestation of the 'sick sinus syndrome' (see Chapter 3).

Postural hypotension

This is an important condition in the elderly and is due to two main causes. Degenerative changes in the autonomic nervous
Autonomic
system that occur with ageing, and especially in diabetics, may result in failure of the normal blood pressure balance with postural changes. Baroreceptor reflexes may be impaired in many conditions, which include diabetic neuropathy, polyneuritis, cerebrovascular disease, Parkinson's disease and high spinal cord blocks as a result of tumours or arterial

94

---

disease. When these baroreceptor mechanisms fail there is resultant inappropriate pooling of blood in the peripheral and visceral veins and this in turn leads to a decreased venous return to the heart and a fall in cardiac output.

Drugs   Drug treatment in the elderly frequently leads to postural hypotension and apart from specific anti-hypertensive agents, it is important to remember that many other drugs may have a significant effect on blood pressure and these include the tricyclic antidepressants, the phenothiazine group, diuretics and alcohol. The question of whether or not to treat measured high blood pressure in the elderly is considered elsewhere (Chapter 2). However, the family physician should be aware of the potential blood-pressure-lowering effects of drugs and in particular, become used to measuring both the sitting and standing blood pressure in elderly subjects.

Electrolytes   Other more unusual causes of postural hypotension should be considered, amongst which electrolyte disturbances, including both hyponatraemia and hypokalaemia and Addison's disease are perhaps the most important. Anaemia and blood loss may also interfere with the older person's ability to adjust to postural changes. Postural hypotension is demonstrated when there is a drop in systolic pressure of 20 mmHg or more between the lying and standing positions. It is useful to measure the blood pressure both after 30 seconds of standing and again after 3 minutes as the postural drop may not occur immediately. The clinical features can vary considerably and may cause nothing more than transient dizziness, whereas in others there may be falling with loss of consciousness. The symptoms are usually worse in the mornings and in particular, may be troublesome if the patient gets out of bed in the middle of the night.

The management of postural hypotension

The management of postural hypotension should include the elimination of all the reversible conditions causing it and giving general advice about rising slowly from the lying or sitting positions. Venous pooling in the legs can be effectively treated by the wearing of supportive bandages or stockings, but these must be correctly applied. Blood volume loss should be replaced by blood or plasma transfusions if this is the problem. When there is no obvious blood loss, or there is hyponatraemia, a sodium-retaining steroid, such as fludrocortisone in a starting dose of 0.1 mg daily orally, may be helpful. This dose can be increased if necessary, provided no significant fluid retention occurs. Vasoconstrictor agents have many side effects and should not be used. Addison's disease can be diagnosed by estimating the serum cortisol levels (see Chapter 13) and giving the patient replacement cortisone. These patients often need a small dose of fludrocortisone as well.

Falls

The most important causes of falls have been discussed in the preceding paragraphs, but there remain some patients who fall repeatedly and who have none of these problems. In many of

Accidental these people the falls are accidental and may result in serious injury. It is essential for the family physician or district nurse to visit the patient's home and to establish that there are no physical reasons for the falls, the commonest being loose mats and wires, slippery floors and steps. All these are particularly dangerous if the patient has any disorder of locomotor function and indeed, the incidence of falls increases with age – about a third of all falls occur in people over the age of 80 years. Patients with Parkinsonism, strokes and osteoarthritis of the hips and knees are greatly at risk if the home circumstances are unsatisfactory and their quality of life can be much improved if the home is well organized. Good lighting, the installation of banisters, grab rails in the bath and lavatory, together with the fixing of loose mats and rugs and the liberal use of non-slip surfaces on the floors and in the bath can make a significant contribution to home safety at minimal expense. These simple manoeuvres can make all the difference between the patient being able to stay in his own home and having to move into more sheltered accommodation. It may often be necessary to call in an expert on the latest home aids and the use of a community or hospital-based occupational therapist for home visiting is an important part of the comprehensive service that should be available to the elderly.

Loss of People who suffer repeated falls at home lose their con-
confidence fidence and may become chair or bed-ridden and, therefore, rehabilitation must be instituted urgently. Referral to an outpatient physiotherapy department or to a geriatric Day Hospital will usually rapidly enable the patient to regain confidence and mobility. In some cases it may be possible to call in a domiciliary physiotherapist if the other services are not readily available.

Table 6.1 Summary of the causes of fits, faints and falls

Epilepsy	
localized	Jacksonian fits
	Temporal lobe fits
generalized	Petit mal fits
	Grand mal fits
Vaso-vagal attacks	Cough syncope
	Micturition syncope
	Carotid sinus hypersensitivity
Postural hypotension	Drugs – antihypertensives, phenothiazines, L-dopa, etc.
	Autonomic nervous system failure
	senile
	diabetes-related
	Electrolyte disturbances
	drugs-related
	Addison's disease
	Blood loss
Vascular causes	Carotid artery stenosis
	Vertebrobasilar insufficiency
	Subclavian steal syndrome
	Aortic valve disease
Cardiac arrhythmias	Heart block ⎫
	Bradycardias ⎬ established or intermittent
	Tachycardias ⎭
Other causes	Accidental falls
	Locomotor instablity
	Parkinson's disease
	strokes
	osteoarthritis

Failing mobility ('gone off his feet' syndrome)

Failing mobility is a very common problem that the family physician meets in the elderly. There are many reasons for loss of mobility and some of these are discussed in the chapter on 'Fits, Faints and Falls'. The majority of the causes of loss of mobility are due to interference with locomotor function, whether this is a result of musculo-skeletal disorder or some neurological impairment. Strokes are an obvious cause of failing mobility and are discussed separately in Chapter 5. In addition to specific diseases interfering with locomotor function, it must be remembered that any illness in the elderly may lead to immobility and that even after the acute illness has been treated successfully the patient may not regain his physical independence. This may be due to lack of drive or loss of confidence, or simply stiffness or 'rustiness' of joints. Thus immobilization should be avoided in the elderly, even during serious illnesses. Rehabilitation should be instituted as soon as possible when patients have 'gone off their feet'.

The problems that lead to failing mobility can be put into three broad categories. There are those with neurological causes, those caused by musculo-skeletal disorders and the

99

problems related to defects of the senses. In this chapter the three categories are treated in that order.

Parkinsonism

Parkinsonism, or the Parkinsonian syndrome, is characterized by:

(1) Tremor,
(2) Rigidity,
(3) Postural abnormalities,
(4) Dyskinesia.

Although paralysis agitans (The Shaking Palsy) was described as long ago as 1817 by James Parkinson it is now clear that there are many other disorders that may produce a similar clinical picture and these include

(1) Drug-induced Parkinsonism,
(2) Post-encephalitic Parkinsonism,
(3) Multi-infarct cerebrovascular disease.

Parkinsonism is a disabling and common disease in the elderly and occurs in about 15 per thousand people over the age of 60 years. Both sexes and all races appear to be affected equally.

The classic description of the 'Shaking Palsy' was a masterpiece of medical writing and James Parkinson's comments and observations are still highly relevant today.

Pathological and biochemical abnormalities

There is loss of the pigmented neurones in the brainstem, mostly in the substantia nigra and its connections and a reduction in the nerve cells in the globus pallidus. Cerebral atrophy tends to occur more frequently in these patients than one would expect for people of similar age.

The substantia nigra projects via the nigro-striatal pathway to the putamen and the caudate nucleus and the neurotransmitter released at its terminals is dopamine. With the loss of neurones in the substantia nigra there is a corresponding reduction in striatal dopamine production. This is not the complete picture of Parkinson's disease since there are also reductions of cerebral noradrenaline and serotonin.

Clinical features

Tremor

This is usually the presenting feature of the disease and is characteristically slow and affects the upper limbs primarily, giving rise to 'pill-rolling' movements of the hands. The legs and head may also be affected. The tremor is present at rest and disappears on movement and is intensified by emotional stress. Although patients are often most embarrassed by the tremor it is not of itself disabling and the other features of the disease are functionally more serious.

Rigidity

Both agonist and antagonist muscles are equally affected and the increase in passive muscular tone is of the 'lead pipe' variety. However, since tremor is usually superimposed upon this, 'cogwheel' rigidity is often found.

Postural abnormalities

Increased rigidity leads to a permanently flexed posture and there is a festinant gait (*'marche a petit pas'*). Posture is also disturbed by the failure to resist a pushing or pulling stress and falls are frequent.

Dyskinesia

In addition to rigidity, there is an inability to initiate movements, both spontaneous and automatic. Thus there is a general poverty of movement, such as a masked face, loss of arm-swinging on walking, loss of blinking, soft monotonous speech and micrographia. These are the features that inconvenience a patient the most and require treatment.

All the above features are present to some degree in Parkinson's disease. However, there are other symptoms and signs that are frequently present and include the following.

Mental disturbances

Although James Parkinson did not describe mental changes in his original essay, there is no doubt that many patients with this condition exhibit intellectual and psychiatric problems. As a result of cerebral atrophy, intellectual impairment is frequently seen in advanced stages of the disease and these patients may be severely demented. Depression, confusional states and frankly psychotic illness with delusions and hallucinations may be seen as the disease progresses.

Gastro-intestinal disturbances

Excessive salivation and dribbling are common in the disease.

Constipation occurs frequently and the majority of patients are unable to maintain their weight.

Drug-induced Parkinsonism

There are several drugs that may induce Parkinsonism, but the most common are the phenothiazine group. Haloperidol (Serenace) is the worst offender in this group and even small doses (1.5 mg daily) may cause significant Parkinsonism. Surprisingly, in much larger doses (20 mg or more daily) this effect does not appear to be a problem. It is wise to give an anti-Parkinsonian drug, such as orphenadrine (Disipal) 50 mg t.d.s. with haloperidol. These drugs tend to inhibit dopamine action in the brain and the Parkinsonian effect may be permanent.

Haloperidol – significance of dose

Post-encephalitic Parkinsonism

This is now rarely seen since the Parkinsonism that followed the pandemics of encephalitis lethargica in the 1920s and 1930s occurred about 10–15 years after the infection.

Multi-infarct cerebrovascular disease

Parkinsonian symptoms are quite common in association with multi-infarct dementia and Alzheimer's disease. In addition to the dementia there are often fits and pyramidal tract signs and these are evidence of widespread brain disease.

Rare causes of Parkinsonism

Progressive supranuclear palsy

This syndrome consists of many features of Parkinsonism together with the loss of conjugate movements of the eyes.

Shy–Drager syndrome

This is a rare condition where the features of Parkinsonism are associated with severe postural hypotension, loss of sweating, headache and sphincter disturbance.

Both these conditions are usually rapidly progressive and are not responsive to anti-Parkinsonian treatment.

Treatment of Parkinsonism

The management of Parkinsonism has been revolutionized by

L-Dopa

102

the introduction of laevodopa treatment. L-Dopa administration increases the level of dopamine in the brain and its effect has been considerably increased and the side-effects reduced by the concurrent use of a decarboxylase inhibitor, which prevents the metabolism of L-dopa to dopamine outside the brain and allows increased replenishment of cerebral dopamine. There are two forms of decarboxylase inhibitor in common use in conjunction with L-dopa, benserazide (Madopar) and carbidopa (Sinemet). L-Dopa treatment does not affect the underlying pathology of the disease and does not interfere with progressive brain damage that is characteristic of Parkinson's disease. Thus there is no indication to use this drug in mildly affected patients.

L-Dopa should always be used with a decarboxylase inhibitor and the choice of compound is largely a matter of personal preference. The decarboxylase inhibitor allows the use of a much smaller dose of L-dopa and so minimizes the unwanted effects of this drug, which are chiefly nausea, vomiting and postural hypotension.

L-Dopa should improve up to 85% of patients with moderate or severe Parkinsonism to some degree, although it is not so effective in the control of the tremor. In the elderly it is best to start with a small dose, such as Madopar 125 mg or Sinemet 110 twice daily and to increase the drugs by one capsule or tablet every other day. Both these preparations are available in larger strengths and patients can be converted to these as necessary to minimize drug-taking. It is wise to spread out the dosage schedules to maintain adequate blood levels and these drugs may ultimately be given three or four times a day. This is important if there is the 'on—off' phenomenon, where the patient gets severe swings from immobility to mobility throughout the day owing to fluctuating dopamine levels. This occurs frequently in the more advanced stages of the disease.

If L-dopa with a decarboxylase inhibitor is given in this way the annoying side-effects of nausea and vomiting are minimized. The dose can be increased until a satisfactory improvement is achieved, or until the toxic side-effects of L-dopa, such as oro-glossal dyskinesia (where there are writhing movements of the mouth) appear. The dose can then be reduced by one tablet. In severe cases patients may be prepared to put up with mild oro-glossal dyskinesia in order to achieve maximum mobility.

The titration of the dose of L-dopa to the patient's improvement is sometimes difficult and always requires continual

Problems in geriatric medicine

supervision. It is often necessary to reduce the dose of L-dopa after a few months, since its effect tends to be cumulative. If the dose of L-dopa is insufficient to control the major symptoms of the disease, it can be given in conjunction with either amantidine or an anti-cholinergic drug (see below).

Bromocriptine

In patients with moderate or severe disease an L-dopa preparation should be used as the treatment of first choice. It is now possible to use bromocriptine (Parlodel) in place of L-dopa if patients cannot tolerate the drug or are troubled by the 'on–off' phenomenon, since bromocriptine, which is a dopamine agonist, appears to have less side-effects and is longer-acting than L-dopa.

Amantidine

Amantidine (Symmetrel) was first introduced as an anti-viral agent, but it has a useful anti-Parkinsonian effect in some patients. Because it has few side-effects it is well worth trying it alone in mild cases or in combination with L-dopa in severe cases. Its action is as yet unexplained, but it can be started in a dose of 100 mg daily and increased to 300 mg daily in divided doses. It may cause nausea, ankle oedema or a confusional state.

Anticholinergic drugs

Until the introduction of L-dopa the anti-cholinergic drugs were the mainstay of treatment for Parkinsonism. These drugs are still of great value and include agents such as orphenadrine (Disipal), benzhexol (Artane), benztropine (Cogentin) and procyclidine (Kemadrin). For mild cases of Parkinsonism, or in combination with the phenothiazine drugs, the anti-cholinergic agents are the treatment of choice. These drugs are especially useful in reducing the excess salivation and to a lesser extent in controlling rigidity. They are not often effective in controlling the tremor of Parkinson's disease. All these drugs are liable to cause unwanted effects, such as dry mouth, urinary retention and confusional states (especially benzhexol) in the elderly. They may all be given in combination with L-dopa in moderate and severe cases.

Drug treatment of Parkinsonism is only one aspect of management of afflicted patients. Counselling of both patient and relatives is most important and the family physician is in an ideal situation to do this. Physiotherapy and occupational therapy, if necessary in a Day Hospital, are essential in the management of this progressive and sometimes longlasting, condition. Referral of the patient to a local expert in this disease, be he physician in geriatrics, neurologist or rehabilitation consultant, may often be of benefit to the patient and useful support to the family physician.

104

Table 7.1 Drug treatment of Parkinsonism

Drug	Indication	Problems
L-Dopa + decarboxylase inhibitor	Moderate to severe Parkinsonism	'On–off' phenomenon, dyskinesias, nausea and vomiting
Bromocriptine	Severe Parkinsonism, 'on–off' phenomenon with L-dopa and intolerance of L-dopa	
Amantidine	Mild Parkinsonism, in association with other drugs in severe Parkinsonism	Nausea, ankle oedema and confusion
Anti-cholinergic agents	Mild to moderate Parkinsonism, in association with other drugs in severe Parkinsonism and in cases of excess salivation	Dry mouth and urinary retention

Benign essential tremor (senile tremor)

This condition is usually inherited as an autosomal dominant trait and no obvious biochemical or pathological cause has yet been identified. Although it is about as common as Parkinsonism it does not appear at rest and usually occurs in the hands on maintaining posture. It may appear for the first time in older age and is then known as 'senile tremor'. It does not usually get worse on purposeful movement and does not lead to significant functional disability. It tends to be slowly progressive and may be helped by β-blocking drugs such as propranolol (Inderal) and by alcohol.

Cerebellar ataxia

Lesions, such as tumour or ischaemic cerebrovascular disease, may involve the cerebellar connections. Interference with the blood supply to the brain stem, as occurs in vertebrobasilar insufficiency or cervical spondylosis, may also cause impairment of cerebellar function. The characteristic abnormality here is an intention tremor and nystagmus. The tremor is absent at rest. There may be considerable disturbance of mobility and these patients walk with a staggering gait and tend to fall.

It is important to exclude a cerebellar tumour and expanding lesions in this area may cause raised intracranial pressure, with headache, vomiting and signs of papilloedema. Acoustic neuromas usually present with vestibular symptoms and signs and unilateral deafness. There may be unilateral facial weakness and the corneal reflex on that side may be absent. If there is any doubt about the diagnosis a CAT scan should be arranged.

Cervical spondylosis

Cervical spondylosis is found in many elderly people. In addition to osteophyte formation and disc protrusion there is frequently associated atheromatous change in the vertebrobasilar system. In addition to the symptoms of giddiness, diplopia, dysarthria and intention tremor, there may be other signs such as long tract involvement with spastic weakness of the legs and cervical radiculitis with sensory changes in the hands. Many patients, however, have no symptoms. X-ray changes in the neck are not closely associated with neurological signs and the diagnosis may be suggested by the precipitation of the symptoms by passive flexion, extension and rotation of the neck. Treatment is by fitting a supportive neck collar, which must be fairly rigid and tight-fitting enough to prevent movements of the neck. It should be worn both by night and day. Some patients will find this method of treatment most uncomfortable and will either discard the collar or wear it loosely so that it does not function adequately.

Osteoarthritis

This is the first of the musculo-skeletal problems to be considered and is an exaggerated manifestation of the ageing process in the articular surfaces. At the age of 65 years between 80 and 90% of the population have radiographic changes of osteoarthritis but only about 20% have significant symptoms of pain and immobility. The articular cartilage becomes thickened and distorted and with continued joint movement the damage accelerates with resultant cartilage loss and osteophyte formation. The ligaments become lax and the joints become deformed and less stable. Ultimately the joints are damaged to such an extent that subluxation or fusion may occur. The weight-bearing joints are most commonly involved; the knees, hips, spine and shoulders in that order of frequency. Symptoms usually arise from only one or two joints, even though many others may be involved radiographically. The main problem is pain, both on exercise and rest and mechanical restriction of movement.

Treatment

The articular changes in osteoarthritis are irreversible, but patients can be helped considerably by conservative management. This consists of analgesic drugs such as aspirin or paracetamol, together with active exercises. Physiotherapy has an important part to play in the management of this condition and should be designed to increase the degree of movement in the affected joints and to strengthen the muscles that move them. It is essential to reduce weight in obese patients.

Physiotherapy

In recent years great advances have been made in the surgical management of this problem by means of arthroplasty, and prosthetic replacement of the knee and hip are extremely satisfactory. The main indications for joint replacement are either severe pain at rest or immobility or a combination of both. The age of the patient is of no great consequence and surgery should be considered on the merits of pain or dysfunction alone. Patients should be referred for consideration of surgery before it is too late for the surgery to be of benefit. It is quite wrong for anyone to have been immobile for any length of time before an orthopaedic opinion has been sought, since it may be extremely difficult to rehabilitate the patient after surgery. This subject is discussed in more detail in Chapter 11.

Prosthetic replacement

Rheumatoid arthritis

Rheumatoid arthritis may be a problem in the elderly, both for the pain and incapacity that occurs in long-standing disease, especially in women. The onset of the disease may appear for the first time in later life, when it occurs as frequently in men as it does in women.

Rheumatoid disease, as opposed to osteoarthritis, usually affects the smaller joints; the fingers, wrists, elbows, ankles and shoulders. There is thickening of the synovial membranes with effusions in the joint and wasting and weakness of the surrounding muscles. In the acute phase the joint is actively inflamed with resultant warmth and redness. There is a constitutional disturbance with malaise, fever, anorexia and weight loss. The erythrocyte sedimentation rate is accelerated and there may be some degree of anaemia. The rheumatoid factor (Latex and Rose Waaler) may show a high titre. More rarely there may be non-articular manifestations, such as pleural effusion, fibrosing alveolitis and small vessel arteritis which may lead to gangrenous changes in the fingers and toes. However, despite the sometimes explosive onset of rheumatoid arthritis in the elderly, the disease is usually more benign than in younger patients and the degree of joint deformity is less.

Acute rheumatoid disease in the elderly leads to local pain in and around the affected joints, with varying degrees of immobility and joint dysfunction. The joints are tender, swollen and hot. The pain is aggravated by movement, and is usually worse in the beginning of the day and tends to improve as the day goes by. Stiffness gradually replaces pain as the disease progresses.

In patients with long-standing rheumatoid disease the problems are different and are those of chronic pain, joint immobility and deformity.

Management of rheumatoid arthritis

In the active phase complete rest of the affected joints is essential. The joint should be positioned correctly and plastazote splints may be very helpful, especially if the wrists or knees are affected. A bed cradle will be useful if any part of the lower limbs are involved. In milder cases soluble aspirin in doses of up to 600 mg 4-hourly may be sufficient to control the disease. There are now many non-steroidal anti-inflammatory drugs available. Indomethazine, phenylbutazone, naproxen and diclofenac may be very useful if simple aspirin fails to control the symptoms. Gold treatment with weekly injections of sodium aurothiomalate (Myocrisin) 50 mg may sometimes be helpful in the acute disease.

The place of corticosteroids in the elderly is controversial, but oral prednisolone in initial doses of up to 40 mg daily may be necessary to control the disease. Sometimes there is a place for intra-articular injections of hydrocortisone. Although the steroid drugs cause many side-effects in the elderly, such as osteoporosis, gastro-intestinal bleeding, fluid retention, diabetes mellitus and predispose to overwhelming infections, their use in the acute disease is justifiable if it is severe and unresponsive to other agents. It is, of course, essential to reduce the dosage as soon as possible and to tail these drugs off at the earliest possible moment.

In many cases the management of the patient can be undertaken at home, provided there are the necessary supportive facilities, not only caring family and friends, but also medical, nursing and physiotherapy help available on a regular basis. If these circumstances do not obtain the patient should be transferred to hospital. The correct management in the early phases of this illness is essential if permanent disability and joint deformity are to be prevented.

Once the acute phase of the disease has been satisfactorily treated it is important to start physiotherapy to reinstate mobility and to strengthen the muscles. This can be achieved satisfactorily either in a Day Hospital or by attendance at a hospital physiotherapy department.

For the chronic rheumatoid patient there is no place for longterm steroid treatment. The non-steroidal anti-inflammatory drugs are of great use, but these too have gastro-intestinal side effects and some, especially phenylbutazone, may cause blood dyscrasias. The main problem with these patients is to preserve mobility and many of them will have significant joint deformity. Physiotherapy has a large place in their management. If pain and immobility persist in spite of adequate conservative treatment, there may be a place for joint replacement, especially of the knee.

Table 7.2   Treatment of rheumatoid arthritis

Acute phase	
Rest affected joints	Splints
	Bed cradle
Drugs	Aspirin
	Non-steroidal and inflammatory drugs e.g. indomethazine, phenylbutazone, naproxen and diclofenac
	Gold
	Steroids
Chronic phase	
Physiotherapy	
Non-steroidal and inflammatory drugs	
Mechanical and electrical devices	

It is in the patient with established disability that the family physician and his team have an important part to play. Since the majority of these patients will be women, proper assessment of the home situation is necessary. Routine housework, cooking and shopping may be a real problem. Alterations to fixtures and fittings, especially in the kitchen and bathroom, may be of great assistance and there are now a wide range of mechanical and electrical devices available that may improve the patient's ability to cope adequately at home. An occupational therapist should be involved to help match the home alterations with the patient's needs. The social services department may be able to assist with provision of home helps or meals on wheels. In some cases it may be necessary to rehouse the patient in a bungalow, ground floor apartment or even in a residential home for the elderly and infirm.

Septic arthritis

This condition is especially common in the elderly and may be present with existing rheumatoid arthritis. The importance of recognizing joint sepsis is vital so that the appropriate anti-biotic treatment can be given and the dangerous administration of cortico-steroids may be avoided.

Bacteraemia is not uncommon in the elderly and the source of infection is usually the bowel or the urinary tract. The majority of causative organisms are gram-negative, such as *E. coli*. More rarely the portal of entry may be the gall bladder, the throat or even directly into the joint after injury or aspiration.

The signs are those of an acute mono- or poly-articular inflammation. There may be other obvious signs of bacteraemia or even bacterial endocarditis. It is essential to take blood cultures and to aspirate the affected joint. Treatment is with the appropriate systemic antibiotic and splintage of the joint.

Gout

Gout is the result of the deposition of uric acid crystals in a joint, which causes an acute arthritis. This occurs when the body becomes supersaturated with uric acid owing either to excessive synthesis (as in idiopathic gout, myeloproliferative diseases, reticuloses and chronic haemolytic states), or to diminished excretion of uric acid (diuretic drugs, psoriasis and chronic renal disease), or a combination of both.

The acute disease begins suddenly with arthritis of a single small joint and in about half of the patients this is the first metatarso-phalangeal joint. The pain is extremely severe and there may be a generalized systemic upset. Gradually the joint settles down without residual damage, but, if the disease recurs frequently, the articular cartilage becomes destroyed and the joint deformed. In chronic gout tophi of monosodium urate appear close to joints in the subarticular region of bones, in bursae and tendon sheaths, in the pinna of the ear, the kidneys, eyes or in the heart.

Treatment of gout

The acute attack is best treated with oral phenylbutazone or indomethazine but a single injection of ACTH may be given as well. The xanthine oxidase inhibitor allopurinol (Zyloric) 200–400 mg per day, should be given to all patients with established gout and to those with myeloproliferative diseases. The dose is monitored by measuring the serum uric acid level regularly. Many elderly patients have their gout precipitated by diuretic agents and, if possible, these should be stopped. Dietary control is not all that important, but the patient should be advised to lose weight and to restrict excessive intake of purines. Any of the myeloproliferative disorders may cause gout, but only polycythaemia rubra vera can be effectively controlled (see Chapter 12).

Pseudogout

Pyrophos-phate arthropathy

This is a disease which is increasingly common as age advances. The pathological mechanism is the same as in gout, except that instead of uric acid crystals in the joints there is a deposition of sodium pyrophosphate, which appears as birefringent crystals under polarized light microscopy. The characteristic X-ray finding in this condition is chondrocalcinosis (calcified cartilage), which is most easily seen in the menisci of the knee joints. The same picture may also be seen in the symphysis pubis and the radio-ulnar joint of the wrist. Chondrocalcinosis may not necessarily be associated with pyrophosphate arthropathy and occurs in osteoarthritis, haemochromatosis and hyperparathyroidism. The diagnosis of pyrophosphate arthropathy is confirmed by aspirating synovial fluid and examining it under microscope.

Treatment

Treatment of pseudogout consists of giving adequate doses of non-steroidal anti-inflammatory drugs in the acute attack. Joint effusions should be aspirated.

Other joint disorders causing immobility

Neuropathic joints

Neuropathic arthropathy may occur when there is impairment of pain or joint position sensation. The most frequent cause of this is diabetes mellitus and it is more likely to occur if hyperglycaemia is not controlled. Tabes dorsalis and syringomyelia cause the same problems. Patients who have repeated intra-articular injections of steroids may develop a neuropathic arthropathy. The joints are pain-free and often greatly disorganized, with resultant severe locomotor problems. The knee joint causes the greatest functional impairment.

Malignant diseases

Apart from the myeloproliferative disorders other malignant diseases can involve the joints. Hypertrophic pulmonary osteoarthropathy due to carcinoma of the lung may precede the primary tumour, but rarely causes a problem with mobility. Multiple myeloma may produce amyloid deposition in the small joints and cause a polyarthritis resembling rheumatoid arthritis.

Polymyalgia rheumatica and giant cell arteritis

Polymyalgia rheumatica and giant cell, or cranial, arteritis are diseases of old age and virtually never occur before the age of 60 years. It is now thought that they are variants of the same disease. The cause of these conditions is not understood, but in both there may be giant cell infiltration of the media of the temporal arteries.

Polymyalgia

Characteristically polymyalgia rheumatica presents with pain, stiffness and sometimes tenderness in the shoulder girdle muscles. This may be associated with similar symptoms in the pelvic girdle. The joints are not involved. There is always some systemic upset, with malaise, fever and sweating at night. Immobility is not usually a problem.

Temporal arteritis

Temporal arteritis (giant cell arteritis) is a true panarteritis which affects vessels of all sizes. The temporal arteries are the most commonly involved and produce symptoms of unilateral or bilateral headache with tenderness over the affected vessel. Combing the hair is painful. There may be segmental occlusion of the vessels by thrombosis and intimal proliferation. The retinal artery can be occluded and lead to sudden blindness, but other vessels, especially the coronary, renal and cerebral arteries, may be thrombosed. Sometimes the typical features of polymyalgia rheumatica occur, and there is a generalized systemic upset, with fever and malaise.

Erythrocyte sedimentation rate

The erythrocyte sedimentation rate is always accelerated, often up to 100 mm in the first hour. The serum proteins are abnormal and there is usually an increase in the α_1 and α_2 globulins. All the tests for rheumatoid factor and the immune profile are negative.

Diagnosis

The diagnosis is a clinical one, supported by the appropriate blood tests, i.e. erythrocyte sedimentation rate and serum proteins and preferably, a positive temporal artery biopsy. The response to treatment is highly supportive, since all these patients should respond dramatically to substantial doses of steroids, such as prednisolone 60 mg orally in divided daily doses. As soon as the symptoms subside and the ESR falls, the dose of prednisolone should be progressively reduced to a maintenance level of about 7.5–10 mg daily. Immediate treatment of this condition is essential in order to avoid catastrophic complications of the disease, such as blindness, stroke or myocardial infarction.

Steroid treatment

It used to be taught that polymyalgia rheumatica and giant cell arteritis were self-limiting conditions and that steroid treatment could be tailed-off in between one and two years. Whilst in a minority of cases this is true, many patients will relapse after the steroids are withdrawn and it may be necessary to treat with steroids for many years.

Other musculo-skeletal disorders causing immobility

There are countless other conditions affecting this system that cause immobility and these include fractures, osteomalacia and Paget's disease (see Chapter 11). However, disorders of the shoulder are frequent and important in the elderly since they may cause serious impairment of independence.

Capsulitis of the shoulder

Capsulitis of the shoulder is a common problem in the elderly and may occur spontaneously as well as after trauma, upper limb fractures, hemiplegia and following myocardial infarction. There is an inability to actively elevate the arm and a loss of passive movement of the shoulder joint. In supraspinatus tendinitis a full range of passive shoulder movements are usually retained and unlike capsulitis of the shoulder where it is usually normal, the X-ray may show some calcific deposits in the supraspinatus tendon. The treatment of both these conditions is with physiotherapy and applications of either heat or ice may be helpful. Hydrocortisone injections of the joint may also be useful, if physiotherapy fails to improve the condition.

Supraspinatus tendinitis

Disorders of sight causing immobility

Visual disturbances are extremely common in older age and constitute a major hazard to mobility. The lens becomes increasingly inelastic with age and in the elderly the power of accommodation is lost. This not only interferes with reading, but, if not corrected, will blur near vision and result in the patient

113

bumping into objects that he has not seen clearly. Visual correction is often with bifocal glasses but these themselves may also cause difficulty with seeing hazards such as steps and result in falls.

Cataract
Disabling lens opacity (cataract) occurs in about 5% of the elderly population. In patients with diabetes mellitus the incidence of lens opacity is much greater and tends to occur at a younger age. In early cases the vision is merely misty, but this progresses to increasing loss of visual acuity. At this stage there is inevitable loss of mobility, which is not easily regained when the lens has been extracted owing to the distortion caused by the corrective spectacles.

Glaucoma
Glaucoma and macular degeneration are important causes of visual loss in the elderly. Angle-closure glaucoma presents with pain as well as visual disturbance, but a much greater problem is that of open-angle glaucoma which is of much more insidious onset. In this situation there is often some established field defect before the patient presents to the family physician. It is much more common in myopic people. Glaucoma can be treated medically with pilocarpine eye drops, or surgically by a drainage operation.

Macular degeneration
Macular degeneration is a progressive disease where there is new vessel formation in the region of the macula. On examination there is fine pigmentary stippling around the macula, and there is usually marked loss of vision. In more advanced cases the pigmentation is much heavier and there are surrounding white areas of choroidal atrophy. Treatment is not very satisfactory, but photocoagulation may prevent progression of the early lesions and be of use in the pre-symptomatic phase.

Sudden loss of vision
Sudden loss of vision is not very common, but does occur when there is occlusion of the retinal artery. This may occur in a number of conditions, of which temporal arteritis is the most important (see above). It may also occur with thrombotic or embolic lesions in association with stroke, cartoid artery stenosis or atrial fibrillation. Retinal vein occlusion is rare, but may occur with macroglobulinaemia and polycythaemia. Retinal detachment will cause sudden loss of vision.

Field defect loss
Field defects, such as hemianopia, are common findings after strokes and may cause immobility. Any visual loss will embarrass a patient's mobility and a thorough understanding and assessment of the loss is important. The patient should remain in surroundings that he knows well. White sticks and walking frames help to maintain mobility and confidence. Ob-

114

viously corrective spectacles and operative procedures, such as lens extraction and drainage operations, may be of help in relevant cases and referral should be made early to an ophthalmologist. For those who cannot read, talking books may be of comfort and interest and it may be necessary to reorganize the patient's life-style to cope with the difficulties.

Disorders of the ear contributing to loss of mobility

Deafness may be a serious embarrassment to mobility in the elderly and in many leads to considerable social isolation. Many deaf old people are mentally disturbed. Probably about a third of retired people have significant hearing loss. What is of great concern is that population surveys have suggested that of those who are deaf only about two thirds have actually had any hearing tests.

Presbyacusis Presbyacusis implies changes in the auditory system that are related purely to age, as opposed to those due to pathological problems associated with the ear. With increasing age there is hearing loss for high tones, difficulty in distinguishing tones of different frequencies, difficulty in ascertaining the direction of sound and distortion of the time relationship of sound. Sometimes speech itself may also be impaired.

The management of presbyacusis lies firstly in the correct identification of the problem. Speech audiometry should be performed and some assessment of the effect of background noise on speech intelligibility should ideally be examined. The patient should be referred to a specialist department. Correction is by means of a hearing aid, which is best worn behind the ear, as this is cosmetically most satisfactory and will enable the patient to turn his head toward the sound source. Body-worn aids have the advantage of advertising the fact the patient is deaf, but they are psychologically less acceptable and therefore not always worn and suffer the disadvantage of picking up the noise of clothes rubbing.

Menière's syndrome Menière's syndrome consists of deafness, vertigo and tinnitus. The deafness tends to be progressive and the vertigo paroxysmal. There may be nausea and vomiting. Caloric tests will demonstrate impairment of vestibular function. Patients not only suffer the problems of the deaf, but will be liable to fall and become immobile. Medical treatment can be of great help and in mild cases, where the vertigo is a problem, anti-histamine drugs such as promethazine (Phenergan) may be helpful, but betahistine hydrochloride (Serc) is probably the drug of choice. In severe cases surgical interference may be necessary.

Other causes of immobility

Any acute illness may result in immobility in an elderly patient, and after chest or urinary tract infections there may be impairment of physical independence. The cause of this state is not always simple, but there is often a considerable degree of loss of confidence. It is in these situations that attendence at a Day Hospital may be especially useful.

Other obvious causes of immobility such as stroke and amputation are discussed elsewhere (see Chapters 4 and 11). There are other conditions that will result in patients 'going off their feet' which are often not obvious; silent myocardial infarction and postural hypertension to mention two. It is essential to thoroughly examine these patients and to include the measurement of standing blood pressure and an e.c.g. in the assessment.

Incontinence

Stress incontinence – Senile vaginitis – The prostate – Neurogenic incontinence – The uninhibited bladder – Reflex neurogenic bladder – Atonic bladder – Autonomous bladder – Catheters and appliances – Faecal incontinence

Incontinence of urine, faeces or both is a common and devastating problem in old people. Over a quarter of those aged 65 years and over will be incontinent at some time or other. It is more frequent in women than men. Incontinence may be extremely distressing to both patients and their relatives and friends and may destroy the whole social fabric of existence at home and make it impossible for the patient to continue living in the community. Many patients and sometimes their relatives, regard incontinence as a normal accompaniment to ageing; it is not. *Incontinence is not only abnormal, but is nearly always curable.* Even if it cannot be cured, with proper investigation and management it is always possible to overcome the problem.

Causes   Incontinence in the elderly may be due to urological and gynaecological disorders, which may also be seen in younger patients, but in addition the elderly may lose the important neurological mechanisms by which continence is normally maintained.

Systemic illness   Incontinence of urine may be a transient feature of any systemic illness in the elderly, in the same way as an acute confusional state may be. Thus if an old person develops pneumonia and has associated incontinence, the latter usually settles as the acute illness subsides with treatment.

Incontinence may also occur without any malfunction of the anatomical and physiological mechanisms which control

117

Immobility micturition. For example if people are so immobile that they are confined to a chair or bed for long periods without recourse to assistance, it is not surprising that they will eventually soil themselves. It is, therefore, of paramount importance that disorders of mobility and general health be adequately treated before investigating the secondary manifestation of incontinence and to establish that lavatory facilities and assistance are readily accessible.

Iatrogenic Urinary incontinence is rarely a direct side-effect of drug treatment, although *α*-adrenergic blocking agents have occasionally been implicated by causing relaxation of the urethral sphincter, or anti-cholinergic drugs by leading to retention with overflow in men with pre-existing prostatic hypertrophy. However, some drugs may lead indirectly to failure to control micturition: thus long-acting hypnotics may prevent a person from rising at night to empty his bladder and thus lead to nocturnal incontinence, or powerful diuretic drugs may promote such great and rapid urine production that patients of limited mobility cannot cope with the frequent need to micturate in the right place – the loss of the race between the bladder and the lavatory!

Faecal loading The pressure of a rectum loaded with impacted faeces may also lead to incontinence of urine, as well as faeces, and a rectal examination is essential in the assessment of the incontinent patient. If faecal impaction is present the rectum should be cleared by suppositories, enemata or even manual evacuation before other measures are instituted.

Cystitis Occasionally urinary incontinence may be due to acute cystitis, when there is usually fever, frequency, dysuria and tenderness over the bladder. In any event a mid-stream specimen of urine should be cultured and any significant infection treated. However, incontinence is often associated with other bladder disorders resulting in stasis and infection of residual urine, so that treatment of infection does not always improve the control of micturition.

Approach As in any other disorder, the first step in the management of incontinence consists of taking a full history, including drug therapy and examination. The examination must include inspection of the genitalia and digital exploration of the rectum and prostate. Some specific causes of incontinence are considered below; local disorders of the genito-urinary system are, of course, dissimilar in the sexes, but impairment of neurological control is common to both men and women and will be considered jointly.

118

Stress incontinence

Stress incontinence is a common complaint occurring in
women of all ages. The bladder lies on the muscles of the pelvic
floor, with the urethra normally emerging at a right angle. It is
this angle which constitutes the 'internal sphincter' and is most
important in maintaining continence; the 'external urethral
sphincter' plays little part. If weakness of the pelvic diaphragm
is associated with uterine prolapse the patient may suffer from
stress incontinence. In this condition sharp rises in intra-
abdominal pressure, such as occur in coughing or sneezing,
overcome the weakened internal sphincter and lead to leakage
of small amounts of urine. The history is typical and the
diagnosis may be confirmed by examination, when leakage of
urine on coughing will be seen; a degree of urethrocoele and
cystocoele may also be obvious. Just occasionally a micturating
cystogram must be performed to demonstrate stress incontinence.

Some patients can learn to control the muscles of the
pelvic floor and increase their tone with help of physiotherapy.
When this fails a ring pessary should be tried, or a
gynaecological repair in those who are fit for surgery. A few
elderly patients do not improve with pelvic floor exercises and
a ring pessary and they may not be fit for a repair operation.
Since stress incontinence involves the leakage of only small
amounts of urine, such cases can usually be dealt with by
means of incontinence pads. The most suitable types are either
those worn as a sanitary pad which form a gel on contact with
urine and contain a deodorant, or those in which the pad is inserted into a pouch in a pair of well-fitting 'Kanga Pants'.

Internal sphincter

Management

Senile vaginitis

Both the vagina and the female urethra are lined by stratified
squamous epithelium, which in the elderly may also extend on
to the trigone of the bladder. This epithelium is sensitive to
oestrogens and may become atrophic when hormone levels are
insufficient. The presence of senile vaginitis on examination
implies that there will be a similar urethritis and this may lead
to incontinence. The condition responds well to oestrogens,
either as a locally applied cream or taken orally.

The prostate

In men the bladder outlet may be obstructed by an enlarged
prostate gland, especially the middle lobe. This may be due to

benign prostatic hypertrophy or to a carcinoma. This usually presents as chronic retention with overflow incontinence, preceded by the typical symptoms of prostatism, such as a poor stream and hesitancy. There is also frequency of micturition and nocturia. In this situation the bladder will be distended and palpable in the abdomen, and rectal examination will reveal the size and consistency of the prostate. Occasionally prostatic disease interferes with the internal sphincter and leads to incontinence with a bladder of small volume.

Retention with overflow

Chronic retention with overflow due to prostatic enlargement is best dealt with surgically, usually by transurethral resection of the gland. For prostatic carcinoma causing incontinence, small doses of oestrogens, e.g. stilboestrol 1 mg three times daily, may be helpful. If the patient is not fit for any kind of surgical procedure and this is rare, it is not sufficient to deal with the incontinence with a urinal, since this leaves the bladder distended and allows back-pressure to damage the kidneys. An indwelling silastic catheter must be passed through the site of obstruction. A small proportion of men who have had their prostates resected surgically will remain incontinent; either because of some other pre-existing factor or because the internal sphincter mechanism is damaged at operation.

Neurogenic incontinence

The most frequent cause of incontinence in the elderly is impairment of the neurological mechanisms which control micturition. It is, therefore, necessary to consider how this control operates normally. Essentially, micturition is a reflex action mediated by the sacral parasympathetic nerves which pass to the detrusor muscle of the bladder and respond to increasing stretch as the bladder fills. During childhood control of micturition is acquired as higher inhibitory pathways develop which suppress the bladder contraction until there is a conscious desire to void urine. These inhibitory pathways originate in the frontal cerebral cortex, where sensation of bladder distension is perceived via fibres ascending in the spinal cord and from which fibres return to the sacral region by descending the spinal cord. The ascending and descending pathways are subject to various facilitatory and inhibitory influences as they traverse the brain stem and spinal cord.

It is thus apparent that disruption of these pathways at any level may result in incontinence; if the higher cerebral

Uninhibited bladder

centres do not function normally inhibition of bladder emptying is lost – the 'uninhibited bladder'. If both sensory and motor pathways in the spinal cord are affected the bladder is devoid

of facilitatory or inhibitory input to the sacral reflex arc, which
then operates independently as it does in babies. This is known
as the 'reflex neurogenic bladder'. If only sensory nerves in the
posterior cord are involved, but the motor pathways remain intact, bladder distension is not perceived, the inhibitory in-

fluence of higher centres remains predominant and retention
with overflow incontinence develops – the 'atonic bladder'.
Finally, at the lowest level of control the sacral nerves them-

selves may be damaged, depriving the bladder of all central
influences – the 'autonomous bladder'.

It is also apparent from a consideration of these nervous
pathways that the cholinergic innervation to the bladder
detrusor muscle is open to therapeutic manipulation. Another
site at which drugs may usefully act is the internal sphincter,
contraction of which is effected by α-adrenergic sympathetic
nerves. The presentation and treatment of the various
neurogenic lesions is detailed below; in many cases the diag-

nosis is best established by use of the cystometrogram. This is a
method by which the bladder is filled via a double-lumen
catheter and the pressure response is recorded either
manometrically or by a transducer. It would be a counsel of
perfection for all incontinent patients to be investigated in this
way, but a cystometrogram may be an invaluable help in
management and it is increasingly employed in specialist
geriatric hospitals. Perhaps the most important impact of
cystometry is that its use will improve therapy, both by permit-
ting identification of patients with defined bladder disorders
and as a means of obtaining objective measurements of
response to therapy.

The uninhibited bladder

The uninhibited bladder is the commonest cause of incontinence in the elderly. Cortical inhibitory centres no longer
function, so that bladder detrusor contractions are not sup-
pressed and as the intravesical pressure rises above that ex-
erted by the urethral sphincter, the bladder empties its contents. Although bladder sensation is intact, the contractions
occur without warning so that the first indication a patient
receives of impending incontinence is only a few seconds
before urine appears at the meatus. Thus attempts to control
such incontinence by increasing patient mobility or provision
of bedside commodes or bottles are doomed to failure. Since

the whole bladder contents are voided, absorbent pads cannot cope with the problem satisfactorily. Even frequent regular toiletting is largely unsuccessful as it necessitates constant supervision even during the night and often incontinence occurs between visits to the lavatory.

Causes   The underlying cerebral disease leading to an uninhibited bladder is often senile degeneration and there may be associated intellectual impairment and a tendency to falls. Evidence of cerebrovascular disease with a history of previous strokes is also commonly found. Rarely, focal lesions in the region of the frontal cortex may cause incontinence, such as a parasagittal meningioma. Sometimes there is no obvious lesion within the nervous system and the presentation is slightly different: the uninhibited contraction is triggered by a stimulus such as a cough or rising from a chair. This is known as the

Unstable bladder   'unstable bladder' and is distinguished from stress incontinence by the fact that the whole bladder contents are voided rather than a small leak. On the cystometrogram, filling of the uninhibited bladder results in unsuppressed contraction, the rise in pressure leading to incontinence often when the bladder contains only a small volume. The unstable bladder does not show such contractions until a stimulus such as asking the patient to cough.

Treatment   The treatment of the uninhibited and unstable bladders is by drugs aimed at blocking cholinergic impulses to the detrusor muscle, or direct smooth muscle relaxants. Of the latter, flavoxate is the most commonly prescribed, but there is little evidence for its efficacy. Emepronium bromide is often used as an anti-cholinergic agent, but it is poorly absorbed from the gut and is ineffective in some patients. The most useful drug for the uninhibited bladder is probably imipramine, which has considerable anti-cholinergic properties. It may also be helpful to increase the tone of the urethral sphincter by using adrenergic agonist drugs, for example ephedrine.

Reflex neurogenic bladder

The reflex neurogenic bladder occurs when both motor and sensory tracts in the spinal cord are interrupted, for example as a result of traumatic spinal cord transection or multiple sclerosis. The patient has neither sensation of bladder fullness nor the ability to initiate bladder contraction. The bladder thus fills and empties reflexly; occasional patients can initiate reflex bladder emptying by stimulating the skin also innervated

122

by sacral nerves, but for many there is no alternative to catheterization.

Atonic bladder

This type of overflow incontinence is associated with a painless distended bladder which never empties completely. There may be infection consequent on the large volume of residual urine. Sometimes there is evidence of disease affecting the posterior spinal roots and columns in which bladder sensation travels to the brain, this occurs especially in diabetes mellitus and rarely in tertiary syphilis. It is also important to exclude obstructive lesions of the bladder neck such as prostatic hypertrophy, so that cystoscopy is often a necessary investigation. There remains a group of patients with unexplained atonic bladders, in whom cystometry shows no contractions even when the bladder is filled with two or three litres. Cholinergic agonist drugs, such as carbachol, have been used to stimulate the detrusor muscle, but are not very satisfactory. An alternative approach is to block adrenergic supply to the urethral sphincter with phenoxybenzamine; this is often helpful, though postural hypotension can be a troublesome side effect.

Autonomous bladder

The autonomous bladder is found when the sacral nerves are damaged, for example by spinal artery occlusion or occasionally by a cauda equina tumour. The bladder is denervated and there is accompanying neurological deficit such as loss of sensation in the skin around the anus which is innervated by the same sacral nerves. This is a rare cause of incontinence and can only be dealt with by a catheter or other appliance.

Catheters and appliances

Incontinence pads have already been discussed in the management of stress incontinence. They are of limited value in other types of incontinence because the volume of urine voided is too great to be efficiently absorbed. Various urinals have been developed; none are very effective in females. In males, tubing or sheaths are sometimes used, but are usually unsatisfactory. Many old men are just as wet using such devices because they keep interfering with them or the fitting is not adequate.

Catheterization is a last resort, to be used only when all the measures discussed so far have failed. For some old people, however, a permanent indwelling catheter is more acceptable than constant wetness and may make the difference between remaining in an institution and returning to the community. For longterm use, 'Silastic' self-retaining catheters are most useful and may remain in place for three months or more before needing to be changed. The indications for changing are infected urine or irritation. The catheter should drain into a leg-bag which the patient can empty periodically; a valve prevents retrograde flow of urine from the bag back up the catheter.

It is a common, but ill-advised, practice to culture the urine randomly from longterm catheters and then attempt to eradicate whatever organism is grown. This zeal is misplaced. The urine always becomes infected sooner or later during longterm catheterization and using antibiotics to treat the bacteriological culture simply results in even more resistant organisms. Antibiotics should be reserved for systemic illness in the patient due to such infection, which is rare.

Faecal incontinence

Faecal incontinence is less common than urinary soiling, but is a most unpleasant symptom which can nearly always be treated. The commonest cause is faecal impaction, when faecal and urinary incontinence often coexist. The patient will usually be soiled for most of the time, passing frequent unformed motions (spurious diarrhoea). The diagnosis can be confirmed by rectal examination, though occasionally the rectum appears to be empty and the colon is obstructed with faeces higher up. Some elderly patients have abused purgatives for so long that the autonomic innervation of the colon and rectum is damaged and they are no longer able to move their bowels normally. The first line of treatment is thus to ensure that the bowel is cleared, by means of suppositories, enemata and occasionally manual evacuation. These will have to be administered daily at first and may need to be continued once or twice a week to prevent recurrence of impaction.

Spurious diarrhoea

Diarrhoea in the elderly may result in faecal incontinence. In this case, investigations should be directed towards finding the underlying cause of the diarrhoea and treating the disease responsible. Carcinoma of the large bowel and diverticulitis are common conditions in old people, but ulcerative colitis and Crohn's disease do also occur. Infective diarrhoea or that due

124

to drugs should also be considered. If the patient's general health is otherwise reasonable, diarrhoea should be fully investigated, including sigmoidoscopy and barium studies. Meanwhile, symptomatic relief may be obtained with agents such as codeine phosphate.

Faecal incontinence may also occur as a result of neurological degeneration associated with dementia or cerebrovascular disease, analogous with the uninhibited neurogenic bladder. In this case, the patient passes formed stools once or twice a day into the bed or clothing. It is worth trying to make use of the gastro-colic reflex: some patients can be induced to pass a motion if sat on a lavatory or commode first thing in the morning with a cup of tea. If such measures fail, the only alternative is to keep the patient constipated with drugs such as codeine phospate and empty the bowel once or twice a week with enemata or suppositories.

Summary

Incontinence is a common and distressing symptom in the elderly, which should never be dismissed as a normal part of the normal ageing process. Medical and nursing staff must take a sympathetic and systematic approach to its management. It may be transient and remit as systemic illness is treated. Established incontinence may be due to serious local disease which should be pursued, or due to a simple problem such as faecal impaction. A proper history and an examination which includes the genitalia and the rectum are mandatory; further investigations may also be required. Once the cause of incontinence has been elucidated, an effective means of dealing with the problem can be found in the great majority of cases, even though the symptom may be part of a more general deterioration of the nervous system. The commonest cause of urinary incontinence in the elderly is the uninhibited neurogenic bladder; although simple measures such as improved mobility, regular toiletting and restricting fluid intake before bedtime may have a place in management, ideally drugs must be found which either suppress uninhibited detrusor contractions or keep urethral sphincter pressure above intravesical pressure during contractions. At present, the therapy available is not ideal but imipramine is often effective. The increasing use of cystometry permits more accurate diagnosis in individual cases and will lead to the more rigorous evaluation of drugs in current use and the development of more effective treatments.

Memory, confusion and sleep

Dementia (chronic brain failure) – Senile (primary neuronal) dementia – Natural history of senile dementia – Differential diagnosis of senile dementia – Tests of mental function – Management of dementia – Arteriosclerotic (multi-infarct) dementia – Secondary dementia – Toxic confusional states – Depression – Alcoholism – The Diogenes syndrome – Problems with sleep

Psychiatric disturbances in the elderly will present the family physician with some of his most difficult problems. This is not only because of the great numbers of people involved, but also because of the time and energy that these patients demand of health care. Many studies have indicated that between 4 and 6% of the population over the age of 65 years suffer from definite organic psychiatric disorders. Even within this group the prevalence of psychiatric disease shows a remarkable increase with age. Studies in both England and Scandinavia estimate that 22% of those over 80 years have significant psychiatric disturbance. Perhaps this is not so surprising when one remembers that major neuronal loss in the elderly coincides with loss of status and companionship – often by bereavement, insecurity because of retirement, worry about death and disability, and often failing physical health.

Dementia (chronic brain failure)

Dementia indicates a global loss of intellectual function that is usually irreversible. It is extremely common and affects about

10% of those aged 65 years and over, and about 20% of those over 80 years. The causes of brain failure are numerous and complex and some understanding of the ageing changes in the brain is important.

As age advances the brain tends to atrophy with shrinkage of the gyri and widening of the sulci. This is more marked in the frontal lobes. There is a progressive loss of cerebral neurones after the age of 25 years, but, more importantly, it is the impairment of neurotransmitters associated with cell loss that adversely affects cerebral function. Atherosclerotic changes in the cerebral arterial tree become increasingly apparent as age advances and this will lead to cerebral atrophy. There are other microscopical changes that occur in the brain with age and these include senile plaques and neurofibrillary tangles.

The vast majority of elderly patients with dementia have diseases associated with old age, but a small proportion have so-called 'pre-senile' dementia and have survived into old age.

Pre-senile dementia is rare and is caused by such conditions as Alzheimer's and Pick's disease and Huntington's chorea. All these patients will have symptoms before the age of 65 years. The great majority of dementias occur in people above this age and the main categories are:

Senile (primary neuronal),
Arteriosclerotic (multi-infarct),
Mixed senile and arteriosclerotic,
Secondary (myxoedema, vitamin B_{12} and folate deficiency, etc).

Senile (primary neuronal) dementia

This is the commonest type of dementia and accounts for about 50% of all cases. There is a substantial loss of cerebral neurones and this is associated with thinning of the cortex, widening of the sulci and shrinkage of the gyri. It is still uncertain whether this phenomenon is an exaggerated form of the normal ageing changes or due to a specific disease process. Electron microscopy shows a proliferation of senile plaques and neurofibrillary tangles. Biochemically it can be shown that there is depletion of neurotransmitters and other enzyme changes.

The clinical features of dementia are common to all types and are conveniently summarized here.

Memory loss

The short-term memory is principally affected, whilst distant memory is relatively well preserved, although in advanced cases this is also involved. This represents an exaggeration of the normal memory impairment of ageing, although it is sometimes difficult to draw a line between the two.

Confusion and disorders of behaviour

These are generally secondary to the memory loss. Patients with severe memory loss will forget what the time is, where they are and where they have placed things. In advanced cases they may even forget their own names. All this leads to confusion and anxiety. Patients tend to wander and often get lost. Because they may lose their belongings, paranoid features are common and friends and relatives will constantly be accused of stealing. Patients may become aggressive or, conversely, withdrawn. Socially unacceptable behaviour is common, especially incontinence of urine and faeces. Worse still, patients may urinate and defaecate in totally inappropriate places. Sexual exposure and wandering naked in the street occurs quite frequently in advanced cases.

Intellectual impairment

Intellectual ability becomes progressively impaired. The main problem is the increasing inability to grasp new ideas and to learn. When this is coupled with *the memory loss,* normal conversation with a demented patient becomes more difficult and frustrating for both the normal person and the patient. Thus dements tend to become socially isolated and the behaviour problems increase.

Personality disintegration

Progressive disintegration of the personality is characteristic of dementia. Sometimes in the early stages of the disease there is an exaggeration of the patient's previous personality traits and it is usually the bad features that emerge more strongly. The individual becomes more and more divorced from reality and fails to recognize that he has a problem.

Natural history of senile dementia

Senile dementia is a progressive disease. The life-style

becomes increasingly fragile and the lone patient becomes less able to look after himself. Feeding and washing become less well organized and the appearance more unkempt. Clothes may be worn inappropriately and may be put on in the wrong order. Even if there are friends or relatives at home the social situation may still break down and some form of institutional care often becomes necessary. Removal from his home environment often results in further deterioration and confusion as these patients cannot easily adapt to strange circumstances. Ultimately physical, as well as mental, deterioration occurs and death follows as a result of bronchopneumonia, pressure sores or malnutrition.

Differential diagnosis of senile dementia

Depression

Depression is common in the elderly and may easily be mistaken for dementia. Sometimes the two co-exist. Apathy, memory loss, neglect and incontinence occur in both dementia and depression. Depression tends to be a more acute illness and the memory impairment is more patchy than in dementia. If there are any features suggestive of depression, treatment with anti-depressive drugs is indicated and the response is usually good.

Toxic confusion

Toxic confusional states may sometimes be confused with dementia, but the history in the former is of short duration and usually of acute onset. There is confusion and disorientation, but there is often some clouding of consciousness. There may be considerable fluctuation in both the level of consciousness and the behaviour pattern. Hallucinations may be severe. There is often a fever and other signs of infection. Some biochemical disturbances such as hyper- and hypoglycaemia and uraemia may produce confusional states. With correction of the underlying biochemical disturbance or infection the confusional state rapidly improves, unless there is some underlying degree of dementia.

Psychotic states

Psychotic states, such as paraphrenia, may also have some of the features of dementia, but these patients have no memory impairment and their intellect is preserved.

Tests of mental function

Any test of mental function must be simple; both for the convenience of the family physician and also because demented patients are unable to concentrate on lengthy and complex

Table 9.1 Abbreviated RCP test

1.	Age
2.	Time (to the nearest hour)
3.	Address (for recall at the end of the test) e.g. 42 West Street, Crawley.
4.	Year
5.	Name of local hospital
6.	Recognition of two persons by role not name (doctor, nurse etc.)
7.	Date of birth
8.	Year of First World War (either 1914 or 1918)
9.	Name of present monarch or president
10.	Count backwards from 20 to 1. Then Recall No. 3.

questionnaires. There are many formal tests available, but a convenient one is the modified Royal College of Physicians test.

This test may need to be modified for national or local circumstances, but it basically tests memory and the appreciation of time and space. Plenty of time should be allowed for the answers, which can be included in a general conversation. Since memory and learning are impaired early in dementia, there is no problem in repeating this test at frequent intevals.

Management of dementia

Blood screening
A thorough physical examination and routine screening for blood glucose, urea and electrolytes, blood count, B_{12} and folate, calcium and syphilis serology and thyroid function tests is essential. Some formal assessment of mental function should be undertaken to establish a baseline for monitoring progress.

Discussions with relatives
When the diagnosis is established the relatives must be consulted and told of the likely course of the disease and all that it may entail in terms of care and understanding. It is best if the patient can be kept at home and there is a great deal that the family physician can do to make this possible. Relatives are more likely to be able to cope if they know that the doctor's help is always at hand. Relief for relatives is always possible by using Day Centres or luncheon clubs; it may be possible to admit the patient to a local hospital or home for two or three weeks at a time to allow the family to go away on holiday. Regular visits by the doctor or nurse will not only help to monitor the progress of the disease, but also to reassure the relatives and friends that the professionals are taking an interest

Drug treatment
There is little evidence that any drug treatment will influence the course of the disease. It may, however, be worth

trying the effect of a short course of such drugs as naftidrofuryl (Praxilene) 400 mg daily in divided doses, dihydroergot alkaloids (Hydergine) 4.5 mg daily, or isoxsuprine (Duvadilan) 80 mg daily in divided doses. Occasionally one of these drugs may produce a worthwhile improvement.

Sleep problems — Disturbances of sleep and nocturnal wandering may be improved by giving a short-acting hypnotic, such as chlormethiazole (Heminevrin) 0.5–1.0 g or temazepam (Normison) 10–20 mg at night. If there are problems with behaviour at night which are not controlled by hypnotics alone it is worth adding a phenothiazine drug, such as thioridazine (Melleril) 50–75 mg, or promazine (Sparine) 50–100 mg. Daytime agitation or behaviour problems are best treated with thioridazine or promazine. The use of diazepam (Valium) is widespread, but it has a long half-life and is probably not a good drug to use in the elderly. Alcohol may cause a toxic confusional state in the elderly and is best avoided.

There is, of course, a limit to what one can do in this progressive disease and ultimately it may be necessary to transfer the patient to a home for the elderly mentally infirm or a hospital, either geriatric or psychiatric, depending on the degree of behaviour disorder. Removing the patient from his own environment should always be a last resort but is necessary when the home circumstances begin to break down, for whatever reason.

Arteriosclerotic (multi-infarct) dementia

This type of dementia accounts for about 20% of all cases. It may also co-exist with senile dementia and this probably occurs in the same proportion. The pathological process is basically cerebral arteriosclerosis, but it is more likely to occur with hypertension and may be precipitated by cardiac arrhythmias. As the name implies there are multiple large or small infarcts in the brain and thus there are usually abnormal neurological signs affecting the long tracts (brisk reflexes and extensor plantar responses), the brain stem (dysphagia, dysarthria, palatal and tongue weakness) or other areas of the brain. This dementia may present as transient ischaemic attacks and if the diagnosis is made early it may be possible to modify the course of the disease.

The onset of the illness may be sudden, but is not always so. The first episode is followed by some improvement, but, unless some appropriate treatment is given, a further episode will follow after a variable period. The main difference between this type and senile dementia is the step-wise progress and the marked emotional liability that occurs in the former. The personality tends to be preserved for longer than in senile dementia.

Investigation   The investigation of arteriosclerotic dementia includes a careful neurological examination. Special attention should be paid to the possibility of transient cardiac arrhythmias (see Chapter 3) and an e.c.g. and 24 hour ambulatory d.c.g. should be performed. A careful search for carotid artery bruits should be made. Invasive investigations such as carotid arteriography are not indicated outside neurosurgical centres, but if there is any suspicion of a correctable cardiac or arterial cause the patient should be referred to the relevant specialist.

Treatment

Carotid artery stenosis and cardiac arrhythmias should be treated by any available means (see Chapters 5 and 8). The most frequently found cardiac arrhythmias causing multi-infarct dementia are varying degrees of heart block, sinus node arrest and multiple multifocal ventricular ectopic beats. Sometimes these patients can be greatly helped by the relevant pacemaker implantation or cardio-active drugs. If surgical treatment of carotid artery stenosis is not feasible, or if there is other evidence of generalized vascular disease, carotid endarterectomy is rarely indicated and then there is a place for anticoagulant therapy. This treatment should be for life and unless there is good support for the patient at home, it is better not to embark on anti-coagulants in demented patients because of the difficulty in drug compliance and prothombin time monitoring. There is some evidence that the combination of aspirin 300 mg daily and dipyridamole (Persantin) 100 mg three times daily may be helpful in these cases and the dangers of anticoagulants are avoided.

High blood pressure   The question of lowering high blood pressure in arteriosclerotic dementia is difficult. Many of these patients will have a measured high blood pressure, but one must always remember to take the reading in the standing, as well as in the sitting, position as there may be considerable postural drop (see Chapter 8). Since there is cerebral arteriosclerosis, any reduction in arterial pressure may result in further infarction and it is better not to treat any but the highest levels of blood pressure (e.g. diastolic levels greater than 120 mmHg in the standing position) and when one does so, to lower the pressure very gently by using diuretics first and then, if necessary, β-blocking drugs. There is rarely any place for adrenergic blocking agents such as methyl-dopa.

Secondary dementia

A small proportion of patients have a potentially reversible cause of dementia, such as hyper- and hypothyroidism, vitamin B_{12} and folic acid deficiency, syphilis and tumours, especially a slow-growing meningioma. Unfortunately by the time that the cause of the dementia is found, many of the clinical features are irreversible even if the underlying cause is adequately treated. This is especially true of hypothyroidism (see Chapter 13). The features of dementia are similar to the senile type and stresses the importance of performing a wide battery of tests in anyone who has early signs of brain failure.

Toxic confusional states

Acute toxic confusional states are common in the elderly and it is important that they should be recognized since the treatment is so satisfactory. The main causes are:

> Infections,
> Drugs,
> Metabolic
> Miscellaneous (cardiac, environmental, injury).

Infections   Any infection or fever may give rise to a confusional state, in much the same way as it may in a child. The most common problems occur with chest and urinary tract infections. The very old and frail are most susceptible to confusion and patients with mild degrees of dementia may become suddenly much worse.

Drugs   The elderly are extremely sensitive to drug toxicity and it is they who tend to be given more drugs than any other group. Drug compliance is often very poor in this age group and makes the problem much worse (see Chapter 10). A very large number of drugs may cause confusion, but the chief offenders are barbiturates, alcohol, tranquillizers, phenothiazines and digoxin. Great care must be taken in drug prescribing and a careful search made for old drugs stored up in the patient's home. This subject is discussed more fully in Chapter 10.

Environment
changes

A simple change in the environment may cause confusion, especially if the patient is mildly demented. Any abrupt disturbance in the routine of an elderly person's life may have unexpected and far-reaching effects and should be avoided if at all

Injury

possible. Injuries and operations not only entail removal of the patient from his home but also often involve other factors, such

Diabetes

as an anaesthetic, and special care and understanding is required in these circumstances. Alterations in the normal blood sugar level, either up or down, may cause confusion in any patient, but the elderly are more sensitive to these changes; diabetes mellitus may present in this way, and diabetes re-

Uraemia

quires careful control (see Chapter 13). Uraemia is very common, especially in men with prostatism. Any factor that leads to temporary dehydration may make the uraemia much worse and fluid replacement is essential. Mental disturbance frequently co-exists with myxoedema ('myxoedema madness') and if found in the early stages, will be readily amenable to thyroid replacement (see Chapter 13).

Depression

Depression occurs in as many as 15% of those over 65 years and may be severe. Suicide is a very real risk in these patients and it is important to recognize and treat depression vigorously. The clinical features of depression are well-recognized on the whole and the disease may be endogenous or reactive or a mixture of both. It is easy to recognize the obviously depressed, sad and tearful person, but in the elderly depression may present in less obvious ways. Apathy and lack of energy are usually present and there is nearly always some sleep disorder; either of getting off to sleep (reactive) or early waking (endogenous). The appetite may be poor and this can result in

Table 9.2 Differential diagnosis of dementia, depression and toxic confusional state

Signs and symptoms	Dementia	Depression	Toxic confusion
Recent memory loss	+ +	+	−
Progressive course	+ +	−	−
Recent onset	−	+	+ +
Incontinence of urine	+	+ / −	+
Confusion	+ +	−	+ +
Self-neglect	+ +	+	+
Drowsiness	−	−	+
Disturbed thinking	+ +	−	+ +
Hallucination/delusion	−	−	+ +

135

weight loss and constipation, common enough symptoms in elderly people. Depression should always be suspected unless there is another obvious cause for these symptoms. Many depressed old patients are also very anxious and require different management. Similarly demented people may become depressed.

Treatment

Psychotherapy will go a long way to improving many patients with depression precipitated by bereavement, social isolation, removal from their home and loss of status. It is important to spend time with these people, a commodity usually in short supply with the busy family physician and his team. Para-medical staff and voluntary organizations should be called in Day care if necessary. Day centres and luncheon clubs may have a place in the management of these patients primarily to provide a 'baby-minding' function.

If these measures do not have any major benefit, or if the depression is severe, anti-depressant drugs should be used. There are a large number of these agents and each physician will have his favourites. The tricyclic group are probably the most tried and tested in the elderly, but some may cause excessive drowsiness and confusion. Imipramine (Tofranil) 10 mg three times a day and 25 mg at night is a useful drug for most depressives. The dose can be increased if there is no benefit after two to three weeks. Protryptiline (Concordin) in an initial dose of 5 mg three times daily may have a more rapid effect than imipramine. Clomipramine (Anafranil) 5–10 mg three times daily is useful if there is marked emotional lability especially in those with arteriosclerotic dementia. If there is a severe degree of anxiety and agitation, amitryptiline (Trypti-zol) 10–25 mg three times daily and 50 mg at night is probably the drug of choice. It is worth remembering that there have been several reports of serious cardiac arrhythmias occurring in patients on amitryptiline as well as on other tricyclics. The tetracyclic group of drugs, such as mianserin (Bolvidon), is said to be free of the possible cardiac complications of the tricyclics.

In severe cases of depression where there is risk of suicide or marked withdrawal and drowsiness, or in those who do not respond to adequate medical treatment, one must consider ECT, and in these circumstances the patient should be referred to a psychiatrist.

Alcoholism

Alcoholism is much more common in the elderly than is generally recognized. It has been estimated that the incidence in the United Kingdom in those over 65 years is up to 9%. The majority of these patients are women. About half the elderly alcoholics have always been heavy drinkers, but in the rest the drinking habit starts late in life, usually after a bereavement or other social disaster. Some of these people are frankly depressed. As with all alcoholics these patients may be extremely devious about their drinking habits and their means of obtaining alcohol.

The treatment of elderly alcoholics does not differ from that in younger patients; the drug must be withdrawn and treatment given with chlormethiazole (Heminevrin) to prevent tremor and agitation. If the problem is severe, or if the home circumstances are unsatisfactory it may be necessary to admit the patient to hospital to 'dry out'. Any associated disease, such as depression and hypovitaminosis and anaemia must be treated as well. These patients require a lot of sympathy and support if the habit is to be permanently cured.

The Diogenes syndrome

This bizarre syndrome is not uncommon and most family physicians will have such a patient in the practice. The syndrome is characterized by withdrawal from society, living in extreme squalor, rejecting all forms of medical and social assistance and collecting and hoarding rubbish (syllogomania). It occurs equally in men and women and usually in those of previously good social standing and of moderate to high intelligence. Professional people appear to be particularly prone to this illness. The symptoms start late in life, usually after a bereavement or retirement. There is rarely any major psychiatric disorder, such as depression or paraphrenia, but these patients are very eccentric. They are usually, but not always, known to the physician and to social service organizations as well as neighbours. All help is rejected, and, indeed, it is often difficult to get into their homes because of the mountains of rubbish blocking up the doors and windows! The presentation to the doctor is usually in the form of a severe illness, often a stroke or pneumonia, accompanied by other problems such as deficiency states and anaemia. In women the mortality rate is very high (up to 60%). Hospital admission is usually necessary; compulsory removal under a Court order may be indicated if there is a health danger to other people. It is essential to protect the individual's freedom of choice. Even if the acute illness is corrected and the patient returned home the relapse rate into squalid circumstances is high because of persistent refusal of help. These houses can always be recognized from the outside by pealing and filthy paintwork, broken windows and unkempt gardens. The squalor inside is usually even worse.

Problems with sleep

Disorders of sleep are common as age advances. Electrophysiological studies have now shown that sleep patterns vary at different stages of life. Disordered sleep not only occurs in disease, such as depression and anxiety states, but may be said to be a 'normal' phenomenon of ageing. In the elderly sleep becomes markedly fragmented. It takes longer to go off to sleep and the 'slow wave' sleep is much reduced, with the result that waking during the night will be much more frequent and for longer periods in an older person than in the young. Thus nocturnal sleep will be shorter, but some compensation for this will be made by daytime naps. Conversely, daytime naps may make going off to sleep even more difficult and may even lead to a reversal of the normal diurnal rhythm of sleep. Expectation of sleep also plays a role in the sleep problems of the elderly: after a lifetime of comparative ease in falling to sleep and remaining asleep the elderly person will find himself with difficulties. Sleep which for many years came naturally no longer does so and people who have always slept for seven or eight hours without interruption may think that anything less is abnormal.

Drug dependency

Thus the family physician will frequently be consulted by the elderly about sleep problems. Many old people will demand hypnotic drugs and become dependent on them, especially the barbiturates. In many cases this is both unnecessary and undesirable. A simple explanation of the normal age-related changes in sleep, coupled with reassurance, may well be sufficient to alleviate the patient's worry over not sleeping properly.

Disordered sleep is an important sign of both depression and anxiety and it is necessary to differentiate between the true early morning waking of endogenous depression and age-related changes. It is important not to overlook this sort of sleep disturbance since the treatment of depression will alleviate many of the patient's problems.

If the physician feels it necessary to give hypnotic drugs it is important to choose the right one. Many of the available hypnotics have a long half-life, especially in the elderly, which will then produce problems with hang-over effect, nightmares and confusion. The barbiturates, nitrazepam (Mogadon) and diazepam (Valium) are examples of relatively long-acting drugs and they should not be used as hypnotics in the elderly. The most useful hypnotics for older patients are dichloralphenazone (Welldorm) 650–1300 mg, temazepam (Normison) 10–20 mg, and chlormethiazole (Heminevrin) 500–1000 mg at night. For patients with depression it may be sufficient to give a drug such as amitriptyline (Tryptizol) 50 mg at night but they may need a hypnotic as well. For demented patients with behaviour problems it may be necessary to give a phenothiazine such as promazine (Sparine) 50–100 mg with the hypnotic.

Proper evaluation of sleep patterns in the elderly patient, together with an understanding of the age-related changes in sleep, is a fruitful exercise. Appropriate treatment of disordered sleep will relieve a lot of suffering and anxiety.

Summary

Mental disorders are extremely common and important in the elderly. Dementia is a major problem and occurs in at least 10% of those over 65 years. It is most frequently due to the senile type, treatment of which is far from satisfactory. The arteriosclerotic and secondary forms of dementia may be more amenable to treatment if they are diagnosed early. There is progressive memory impairment for short-term events, confusion and behaviour problems, impairment of the intellect and disintegration of the personality. Dementia may co-exist with depression or a toxic confusional state, either of which should be identified and treated. Proper examination and blood screening is important in these patients so that potentially treatable conditions can be dealt with early.

Depression is frequently seen and may be reactive or endogenous. Sometimes it may present in an atypical way and be missed for some time. Treatment with psychotherapy and drugs is usually very satisfactory. Alcoholism may occur as a symptom of depression and is aggravated, like so many disorders in the elderly, by social isolation and loss of status. Confusional states may be due to infections, drugs, metabolic disturbances, operations and injury. Treatment should be started promptly and the results are gratifying.

Psychotropic drugs should be used with considerable care in the elderly and this applies particularly to tranquillizers and hypnotics. Only those agents with a short half-life should be used.

10 The use and misuse of drug treatment

Drug handling in the elderly – Drug prescribing – Comments on frequently-used drugs – Antirheumatic agents

The elderly have benefited at least as much as patients of all ages from the introduction of powerful modern medications. However, the availability of these effective drugs has brought with it considerable problems for the elderly patient, most particularly in toxic and unwanted side-effects, overdosage and poor compliance. It is now realized that the handling of many drugs in the body is less efficient than in younger people due to the ageing processes and chronic diseases that occur in the elderly. The drug effect on the target organ, especially the brain, may also be altered as a result of age. Perhaps the greatest problem in the elderly is the frequent failure of drug compliance, resulting in either overdosage or inadequate blood levels of prescribed drugs.

Drug handling in the elderly

Absorption

Although malabsorption is not uncommon in the elderly, usually as a result of ischaemic gut disease or previous gastrectomy, its effect on drug absorption is probably not of major importance and in any case may be balanced by diminished metabolism and excretion (see below). The frequent reduction of serum albumin levels that is found in the elderly, may be of significance in the transport of some drugs that are closely bound to albumin, and result in high free levels of agents such as aspirin and phenylbutazone.

141

Metabolism

Liver function The decline in efficiency of liver function in the elderly may lead to an increase in both the level and duration in the blood stream of drugs that are metabolized purely in the liver, such as paracetamol and phenylbutazone. There is obviously great individual variation, but the plasma half-life of some of these substances may be at least 20% longer in elderly patients.

To a much lesser extent, metabolism of drugs may occur in the plasma, gastro-intestinal tract, kidneys and lungs. Reduction of function of these organs as a result of ageing processes therefore may also result in extended plasma half-life of some drugs.

Although metabolism of drugs usually leads to deactivation and loss of pharmacological activity, this is not always so. In some cases, especially with the tricyclic agents and chloral hydrate, the metabolite of the parent drug is responsible for the pharmacological activity and conversely the drug effect in these instances may be diminished in the elderly.

Excretion

Drugs may be excreted from the body either unchanged or as metabolites. The great majority of drugs are excreted in the bile or the urine. Agents that are bound to albumin are generally removed in the proximal renal tubule, and those that are not protein-bound are excreted in either the proximal tubule or through glomerular filtration.

Renal function Renal function diminishes with ageing due to progressive nephron loss. This fact may not be obviously demonstrable by the rather coarse methods that are generally used to assess renal function, such as blood urea and creatinine estimations. The kidney is the sole route of elimination for many drugs, such as digoxin and most antibiotics, and the ageing process has profound implications on the blood levels of such agents. For example, doses of digoxin need to be at least halved in the elderly compared with the young, and daily maintenance doses of 0.0625 mg are usually adequate to maintain therapeutic plasma levels even when the blood urea estimation is normal.

Plasma-binding The therapeutic activity of drugs depends on the degree of plasma-binding and interference with renal function may seriously reduce the albumin-binding of drugs such as phenytoin and the sulphonamides. Quantitative changes in serum albumin may also be associated with renal impairment, as in the nephrotic syndrome, as well as occurring with malnutrition, malabsorption and liver diseases.

Target organ sensitivity

Changes in the sensitivity of receptor sites, especially in the brain, may result in abnormal drug effects in the elderly. Nitra-zepam, a commonly used hypnotic agent, may have more powerful effects on the ageing brain and cause confusion despite 'normal' plasma levels. Phenothiazine drugs are much more likely to cause Parkinsonism and postural hypotension in older patients compared with the young. Deterioration of the autonomic nervous system with age is likely to potentiate the

Table 10.1 Drug interaction

Drug A	Drug B	Result of interaction
Phenytoin	Isoniazid Dicoumarol Chloramphenicol	Increased toxicity of drug A
Tolbutamide	Phenylbutazone Chloramphenicol Dicoumarol	Drug B potentiates drug A Hypoglycaemia
Tolbutamide	Alcohol	Loss of diabetic control
Steroids	Barbiturates Phenytoin Rifampicin	Reduced effect of drug A
Warfarin	Alcohol Barbiturates Dichloralphenazone Carbamazepine Phenytoin	Haemorrhage when drug B is stopped Reduced anticoagulant effect when drugs A and B are given together
MAOI agents	Ephedrine Tyramine (e.g. cheese)	Hypertensive crisis
Digoxin	Carbenoxolone Steroids	Hypokalaemia and digoxin toxicity
Laevodopa	Pyridoxine	Antagonism and loss of effect of A
Cephaloridine	Frusemide	Increased nephrotoxicity of A
Acetohexamide Chlorpropamide	Phenylbutazone	Drug B potentiates drug A Hypoglycaemia
Guanethidine Debrisoquine Bethanidine	Tricyclics Chlorpromazine	Antihypertensive effect of A blocked

hypotensive effect of drugs such as methyldopa and guanethidine and certainly accounts for the marked hypothermic effects of the phenothiazine agents.

Drug interaction

Drug interactions are a problem for the physician dealing with patients of any age, but in the elderly the problems are greater because of the large number of drugs that are often prescribed for multiple disease processes. The mechanisms of drug interaction are extremely complex and often poorly understood, but the more common interactions are listed in Table 10.1.

In addition to interaction between two apparently unrelated drugs, there are two other important points to remember. There may be interaction between drugs acting on the same physiological system and this fact may be used to therapeutic advantage, for example when two antihypertensive agents can be used together to produce a synergistic effect on lowering the blood pressure and similarly when two diuretics such as a thiazide and amiloride are used together to increase the diuretic effect and to prevent potassium loss.

The second point is that the risk of toxicity is increased if drugs with similar toxic effects are used together, for example combinations of nephrotoxic drugs, such as some antibiotics and ototoxic agents such as the aminoglycoside antibiotics and ethercrynic acid.

Secondary effects of drugs

Indirect effects of drugs are important in the elderly since frequently latent disease may be uncovered by their action. Diabetes mellitus may be precipitated by both steroid agents and thiazide diuretics; gout can also be caused by some diuretic agents. Steroids may allow reactivation of healed tuberculosis by decalcification of a healed focus as well as causing osteoporosis. Over-enthusiastic treatment of myxoedema with thyroxine may precipitate heart failure or myocardial infarction. Retention of urine may be caused by the anticholinergic effects of such drugs as the tricyclic antidepressants and antiarrhythmic drugs, such as disopyramide.

Drug prescribing

Short-term

A full and careful assessment of the patient is essential. No

144

Co-operation
cards

drug should be prescribed unless there is a clear indication for it. There should be some assessment of the patient's renal and hepatic function and a thorough knowledge of the toxic and cumulative effects of the drug to be prescribed. It is vital to know exactly what drugs the patient is already taking, and it is very useful to use drug co-operation cards, which clearly state the dosage of the drug, times of taking it, as well as the date of starting and finishing the course. This is especially important if more than one doctor is involved in the patient's management. If the patient is seen at home it is very worthwhile to inspect the bedroom and bathroom for bottles of drugs – one frequently gets alarming surprises!

Drug prescribing should be as simple as possible, both in the number of drugs used and the frequency of administration. There are now many sustained-release agents available and these should be used in preference to multiple dose preparations. The problems of drug interaction should be recognized and combinations of drugs used very carefully.

Compliance

The physical and mental capabilities of the elderly patient and any relatives are extremely relevant. There is no point in prescribing active drugs if they will be taken erroneously or intermittently because of poor compliance. Similarly, the packaging of drugs is important for patients with locomotor or arthritic problems, since it may be difficult for them to physically administer the preparation. Blindness may be a problem, especially if the patient is a diabetic and taking insulin. Wherever possible relatives and friends should be called in to help with drug administration, but it is then important to explain carefully to them the rationale and dosage of the treatment.

Longterm

The main problem with longterm drug treatment is overmedication. Repeat prescriptions should never be given to the elderly without clinical reassessment and review of the co-operation card. Patients frequently amass not only large numbers of different medications but often have several bottles containing the same drug. This leads to overdosage and drug interaction. The proof of this statement is the frequent improvement in the patient's condition when all medication is withdrawn. Where it is possible to monitor the serum levels of a drug, such as with phenobarbitone and epanutin, many instances of overdosage and toxicity can be avoided.

145

Comments on frequently-used drugs

Diuretics

The diuretic agents are some of the most commonly prescribed drugs in the elderly, although their use is often inappropriate. Before discussing the large number of diuretic agents available it will be useful to briefly review the clinical indications for diuretic therapy.

Fluid retention   The main indication for diuretic therapy is the presence of fluid retention, which is most commonly due to cardiac failure, nephrotic syndrome, liver disease and the hypoproteinaemia due to malnutrition or malabsorption. Diuretic agents are also used in the treatment of raised arterial blood pressure and this is discussed in Chapter 2. More rarely diuretics are used in the management of acute poisoning and to achieve reduction in intra-cranial pressure after head injuries. Perhaps the most frequent use of diuretics is in the treatment of swollen legs when they are not due to any of the above causes and this is discussed in Chapter 2.

Benzothiadiazine group of diuretics

These drugs are of moderate activity and are the most widely used types of diuretic agent. The group includes chlorothiazide (Saluric), hydrochlorothiazide (Hydrosaluric) and bendrofluazide (Navidrex). All these drugs are available with combined potassium supplements and although there is some evidence that potassium supplementation is unnecessary in younger patients, it is wise to give them to the elderly, where the diet may be deficient in potassium, especially if there is cardiac failure. Since these drugs are often used in conjunction with digitalis, potassium supplements are even more important since digitalis toxicity is enhanced by hypokalaemia.

Diabetes   The thiazide drugs all interfere with glucose metabolism and may unmask latent diabetes mellitus. They also cause some degree of uric acid retention and may precipitate an attack of

Gout   gout, especially when there is a history of gout or an associated illness causing a high turnover of nucleic acid and overproduction of purines, such as chronic leukaemia.

The benzothiadiazine group of drugs are extremely useful and generally have a diuretic action of up to 24 hours.

Chlorthalidone (Hygroton) is a sulphonamide derivative, but acts in a similar way to the thiazide group. It produces a more prolonged diuresis lasting up to 48 hours and this may be

146

useful if there is incontinence due to prostatism or impaired locomotion.

Potassium-sparing diuretics

Spironolactone (Aldactone) inhibits the effect of aldosterone. It prevents the excretion of potassium and can usefully be given in combination with powerful potassium-losing diuretics. It is especially useful in treating the oedema due to liver disease. It is now available in 100 mg tablets which enables once daily administration.

Amiloride (Midamor) and triamterene (Dytac) also prevent potassium excretion. Both these drugs may be given in combination with a thiazide diuretic, as in hydrochlorothiazide 25 mg and triamterene 50 mg (Dyazide) and hydrochlorothiazide 50 mg and amiloride 5 mg (Moduretic). These drugs act over a period of 24 hours and are very useful in the elderly patient.

Powerful diuretics

Frusemide (Lasix), ethacrynic acid (Edecrin) and bumetanide (Burinex) are the most powerful diuretics available and have a rapid action lasting up to six hours. For extremely rapid effect frusemide 40–160 mg or bumetanide 1–2 mg can be given intravenously. These drugs can be diabetogenic, but their greatest disadvantage in the elderly is accidental incontinence in those who cannot get to the lavatory in time. They also cause potassium loss and should be given with potassium supplements or spironolactone.

Psychotropic drugs

Hypnotics

Sleep disturbance is very common in the elderly and is associated with mental and physical illness and social stress. It is important to isolate the cause of insomnia and remove it, if possible, since purely symptomatic hypnotic prescription rarely induces restful sleep. If hypnotic drugs have to be used it is best to give simple preparations such as chloral hydrate or dichloralphenazone (Welldorm) which can also be given as an elixir. If more modern drugs are to be used temazepam (Normison) 10–20 mg is useful because it has a short halflife. Nitrazepam (Mogadon) may be used, but it sometimes causes confusion and a 'hang-over' effect in the elderly. The barbiturates should never be used.

Tranquillizers

Agitated states are very common in the elderly and the object of the tranquillizers is to damp down psychomotor restlessness and anxiety without inducing sleep. There are two main groups of anxiolytic drugs; the phenothiazines and the benzodiazepines. The phenothiazine group are probably more useful in the elderly and thioridazine (Melleril), promazine (Sparine) and chlorpromazine (Largactil) are the most commonly used, especially if there are hallucinations and delusions accompanying the agitation. All these drugs have anticholinergic, anti-adrenaline and antihistamine effects as well as potentiating the effect of hypnotic agents. Thioridazine in divided doses of 30–300 mg daily is the best choice for elderly ambulant patients and is least likely to produce the side effects of this group, namely photosensitivity, excess lethargy, postural hypotension, constipation, dyskinesia and jaundice. For the very disturbed patient haloperidol (Serenace) in a starting dose of 0.5 mg thrice daily is the most useful drug, but it is likely to cause significant Parkinsonism, though surprisingly, in larger doses (10–15 mg per day), the dyskinetic effect seems to wear off. It is advisable to use an antirigidity agent such as orphenadrine (Disipal) 50 mg thrice daily with haloperidol. Haloperidol is also available as a clear, tasteless liquid, which can be given in a drink for difficult patients. The benzodiazepines are frequently used in the elderly and diazepam (Valium) is as good as any. However, these drugs do cause some sedation and may upset the normal diurnal rhythm of sleep. They may also cause confusion in the elderly. Diazepam is the treatment of choice for status epilepticus given intravenously in a dose of 10 mg. It may also be used to reduce limb spasticity.

Antidepressants

Depression is often a great problem in the elderly and although it is often endogenous it may also be caused by drugs such as reserpine and its derivatives, phenothiazines and β-blocking agents. In the elderly there is no place in family practice for the monoamine oxidase inhibitors and the only antidepressant drugs that should be used are the tricyclic or tetracyclic groups. The tricyclic group have been long-established and the choice of drug is mainly of individual taste; however, some such as amitriptyline (Tryptizol) have a sedative effect as opposed to others such as imipramine (Tofranil) and protryptaline (Concordin) which have more of a stimulant effect. The

148

starting dose of all these drugs should be small and amitriptyline is usefully given at night. Many of this group may not have
significant effects for some time (four to six weeks); however,
after this time a psychiatric opinion should be sought if there is
no improvement. It is important to remember the frequent unwanted effects of these drugs, such as excessive lethargy or
agitation, urinary retention and less commonly, cardiac
arrhythmias. It is thought that the tetracyclic group, such as
mianserin (Norval), are less likely to have effects on the heart.

Cardioactive drugs

Digitalis

Although this drug has been in use for over 200 years in
clinical practice it is very unlikely if it were to be introduced now that it would pass the criteria of the FDA in the
United States or the CSM in the United Kingdom since there is
little margin between the toxic and therapeutic doses. In the
elderly the use of this drug should be severely restricted. Even
though the bioavailability of digoxin (the most commonly used
of the cardiac glycosides) preparations has been standardized,
the plasma levels in the elderly vary considerably with differ-

Renal
impairment

ent dosages. Since digoxin is excreted almost totally in the kidney we can see why the dosage for the elderly is so difficult.
With age there is a reduction in functioning nephrons and
although renal function may appear to be normal on the crude
methods of assessing it clinically, the elderly kidney is unable
to remove digoxin very effectively. It is also known that digoxin
toxicity is increased in the presence of hypokalaemia and this

Potassium

may itself be a problem in the elderly patient taking diuretic
therapy (see above). The principal indication for starting digoxin therapy should be uncontrolled ventricular rates in
association with atrial fibrillation. When the atrial fibrillation
is controlled it may well be possible in many cases to gradually
withdraw digoxin therapy. Cardiac failure in the absence of
atrial fibrillation is not necessarily an indication for digoxin
administration, unless the powerful diuretic agents fail to
control it. Digoxin should be used with especial care after
acute myocardial infarction.

If digoxin has to be used in an elderly patient, then 2 mg in
the first 48 hours is usually an adequate loading dose if renal
function appears to be normal. For maintenance 0.0625 mg
daily will be adequate for most patients over the age of 70
years.

Toxic effects

The toxic effects of digoxin in the elderly are often difficult to recognize, since nausea and vomiting are surprisingly uncommon and serious cardiac arrhythmias and conduction abnormalities are often the first sign of toxicity. The electrocardiogram is the most useful tool to detect digoxin poisoning. The earliest signs are usually first degree A–V nodal block with a prolonged P–R interval and multifocal ventricular ectopic beats (see Chapter 3). With more serious degrees of toxicity virtually any cardiac arrhythmia may appear and second and third degree heart block may be present. There is usually some abnormality of the S–T segment in digoxin toxicity, but this is sometimes difficult to assess in the presence of ischaemic heart disease or left ventricular hypertrophy.

β-blocking drugs

The introduction of drugs that effectively block the β-adrenergic sympathetic receptor nerves in the 1960s was a major therapeutic advance. The indications for these drugs are the same at all age groups and they are extremely useful in the management of many conditions in the elderly. Their chief use is in the control of cardiac arrhythmias, especially the tachycardias associated with thyrotoxicosis, and in the management of patients with significant arterial hypertension and angina (see Chapter 4). These drugs are also useful in the control of senile tremor and have some anxiolytic action.

Peripheral coldness

There are many β-blocking agents available and there may not be great therapeutic advantage in using the newer more cardio-selective drugs such as atenolol (Tenormin) and metoprolol (Lopressor, Betaloc) rather than the older agents such as propranolol (Inderal) and oxprenolol (Trasicor). The main side-effects of the β-blockers in the elderly are peripheral coldness and worsening of peripheral vascular disease. These drugs should also be avoided in patients with obstructive airways disease. Much more rarely there may be disturbance of glucose metabolism and excessive fatigue.

Bradycardia

The dosage of these drugs needs to be titrated to control the symptoms that are being treated. There is no reason why very high doses of these drugs should not be used in the elderly and the bradycardia that they may produce need cause no concern unless it is very severe and causes symptoms. There may be some advantage of using longer-acting preparations of propranolol or oxprenolol (Inderal LA or Slow Trasicor) to simplify drug-taking.

150

Antirheumatic agents

Because musculoskeletal problems are so common in the elderly, often as a result of osteo- or rheumatoid arthritis, these drugs are used very frequently. The management of arthritic problems is discussed in Chapter 7, but because of their frequency of use the unwanted effects of antirheumatic drugs are stressed again here.

Simple aspirin is still probably as effective as any of the newer agents, although in effective doses, at least 4 g daily, it may be poorly tolerated. Aspirin may quite frequently cause epigastric pain and nausea and vomiting. It also causes occult gastrointestinal bleeding and this may occasionally be severe. In high dosage it will cause tinnitus and at all doses it may cause rashes and loss of platelet stickiness. Nevertheless, it is worth trying this drug before the newer preparations.

Gastro-intestinal bleeding

Indomethazine (Indocid) and phenylbutazone (Butazolidine) are also effective anti-inflammatory agents, but again are the

Table 10.2 Problems in drug prescribing

Keep drug prescriptions and regimes as simple and as few as possible.	
Beware of repeat prescriptions.	
Make use of drug co-operation cards.	
Impaired handling of drugs:	
Absorption:	Low plasma albumin and plasma binding
	Phenytoin
	Sulphonamides etc.
Metabolism:	Liver dysfunction
	Paracetamol
	Phenylbutazone etc.
Excretion:	Renal dysfunction
	Digoxin etc.
Target organ sensitivity	
Brain:	Nitrazepam
	Phenothiazines
Autonomic nervous system:	Methyldopa
	Phenothiazines
Drug interaction	
Tolbutamide:	Phenylbutazone
Laevodopa:	Pyridoxine
Warfarin:	Dichloralphenazone
(See Table 10.1)	
Secondary effects of drugs	
Glucose intolerance:	Steroids
	Diuretics
Urinary retention:	Anticholinergics
Handle drugs with care.	

source of considerable side-effects. These are similar to aspirin with the addition that phenylbutazone may rarely cause aplastic anaemia. The use of indomethazine suppositories only reduces the side effects and may be an unacceptable route of administration to many elderly patients.

The proprionic acid derivatives for example, naproxen (Naprosyn), ketoprofen (Orudis, Alrheumat), ibuprofen (Brufen) and dicolfenac (Voltarol), all have gastrointestinal side effects in varying degree. The choice of agent is one best left to physician and patient.

11 Bone disease and fractures

Osteoporosis – Osteomalacia – Paget's disease of bone (osteitis deformans) – Malignant deposits in bone – Fractures

Problems related to ageing changes and pathological diseases of bone, together with the fractures that frequently accompany these, are encountered increasingly by the physician in family practice. In recent years great advances have been made, both in the understanding of bone disease and in the management and rehabilitation of patients with these problems. It is now possible to modify the symptoms and functional incapacity to a significant degree by medical and, sometimes, by surgical means. Detailed knowledge of bone chemistry, much of it only recently discovered, is unnecessary for the practising physician, but an outline of the biochemical changes in individual disorders will be helpful.

Bone is composed of living cells and a bony matrix of collagen upon which bone salts are deposited. There is a constant replacement of both cancellous and cortical bone throughout life and changes in the reformation and resorption of bone underlie the diseases that may occur in the adult skeleton. The maximum amount of bone in the body occurs in the fourth decade and after the age of about 45 years there is a gradual loss of bone from the skeleton, the rate of loss being faster in women than in men (Figure 11.1). The composition of bone is affected by many factors, including oestrogen levels, the action of parathyroid hormone, calcium and vitamin D intake, corticosteroid levels and, very importantly, immobilization.

Bone loss with age

153

Osteoporosis

In this state the bone is of normal composition but there is too little of it. It may occur in people who have a small bone mass in

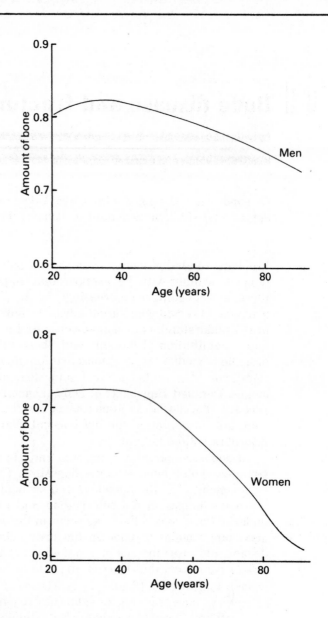

Figure 11.1 Schematic representation of bone loss with age

adult life and who, with advancing years and the normal pattern of bone loss, lose sufficient bone to cause osteoporosis in old age. More frequently there are other factors that cause acceleration of the normal bone loss, and this is seen in post-menopausal women where the reduced oestrogen levels result in increased sensitivity to parathormone and/or vitamin D and result in increased bone resorption and increased calcium requirement. Increased bone loss also occurs when there is corticosteroid excess; this is most often seen in the elderly who are being given steroids for rheumatoid arthritis, asthma, skin diseases and polymyalgia rheumatica. Steroids reduce the intestinal absorption of calcium and probably reduce the tubular resorption of calcium in the kidney. Postmenopausal women are especially sensitive to steroid treatment in this way since there is further depression of oestrogen output by the steroid suppression of the pituitary/adrenal axis.

Osteoporosis occurs when a patient is immobilized, whether by splintage of a fracture, immobility due to stroke or joint disease or due to any of the conditions discussed in Chapter 7. The osteoporosis may be localized, as in a fracture, or generalized when a patient is chair or bedbound. The mechanism of the osteoporosis is probably due to venous stasis and consequent bone resorption. Inadequate calcium intake and absorption is common in the elderly and is especially seen in those who have had a gastrectomy or suffer from intestinal ischaemia. Dietary insufficiency of calcium, especially in male alcoholics, will lead to osteoporosis.

Low calcium intake

Diagnosis

X-ray changes

The diagnosis of osteoporosis in its early stages is difficult and radiological changes are, perhaps, the most useful. Lateral thoracic and lumbar spine X-rays may show vertebral deformation and a lack of contrast between the vertebra and surrounding soft tissues and intervertebral discs. The upper and lower vertebral body margins will be more radio-opaque than the central and it may be possible to see accentuated vertical trabeculation at the expense of the horizontal trabeculae. More advanced stages are characterized by anterior wedging of one or more vertebrae and ultimately the vertebral bodies will become compressed. Biochemical tests are not usually helpful in the diagnosis of osteoporosis, as the plasma calcium and alkaline phosphatase are often within the normal range (see Table 11.1). The urinary calcium and hydroxyproline levels may be raised, but these tests are not specific.

Clinical features

The clinical features of osteoporosis vary from the patient having no symptoms at all, to severe backache and major fractures, for example of the femoral neck. Backache is the com-

Backache monest symptom and may be chronic and severe. It is nearly always much worse on movement, especially rotational movements and is relieved by immobilization. Spinal deformities may occur when there is vertebral wedging and compression. In advanced cases there will be significant loss of height. Thoracic kyphosis may be very severe and lead to extreme respiratory embarrassment. Patients with osteopor-

Fractures osis have an increased liability to fractures of the femoral neck and wrist, but these fractures are common in the elderly age group anyway and may occur for many other reasons, examples of which are osteomalacia and pathological fractures from secondary malignant deposits.

Treatment of osteoporosis

It is important to identify the fast bone losers, whether these be postmenopausal women, those on steroids, or those who start

Calcium elderly life with small bone mass. Oral calcium supplements will help and should be given in a dose of between 800 – 1200 mg per day. If there is evidence of malabsorption of calcium, as in

Vitamin D those on steroid treatment, the administration of vitamin D 50 000 units twice weekly will help. Postmenopausal women with osteoporosis should receive oral vitamin D and cyclical oestrogens, such as ethinyl oestradiol 0.025 mg/day for three weeks out of four. There will be withdrawal bleeding, of which the patient should be warned. Oestrogens should not be given to patients with ischaemic heart disease or a history of thrombo-embolism and given to the over 65s with caution. Nor-ethisterone may be a safer alternative for these people. Sodium fluoride 50 mg daily may be of some use, but the evidence is inconclusive. Anabolic steroids are widely used in the general treatment of osteoporosis, but there is little evidence that they are of use. Radiological and biochemical screening should be undertaken in all patients receiving treatment.

Backache Backache should be treated symptomatically with analgesics, rest and infra-red radiation. However, it should be remember-ed that immobility is a major cause of osteoporosis in the elderly and it is essential to maintain maximum mobility in these pat-ients (see Chapter 7). A recent painful vertebral compression episode may be an exception and should be treated by three weeks bed rest and analgesics.

Osteomalacia

Osteomalacia is a generalized disease of bone and is

characterized by decalcification of the skeleton in which the bony matrix is normal. It is caused by a lack of vitamin D. This is an important and correctable disorder and probably occurs in at least 5% of people over 70 years.

Sources of
vitamin D

The two major sources of vitamin D are dietary and from the action of ultraviolet radiation upon a precursor in the skin.

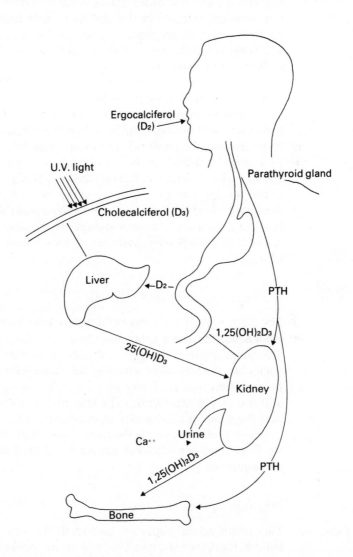

Schematic representation of vitamin D metabolism

Figure 11.2

The dietary vitamin occurs in the form of vitamin D_2 where it is found in fish oil, eggs, milk and cereals. In the United Kingdom margarine is fortified with vitamin D and in the United States milk is also fortified. Thus malabsorption states and obstructive jaundice will lead to dietary vitamin D lack.

Vitamin D_3 is formed in the skin by the action of ultraviolet light. Interference with sunlight through atmospheric pollution will drastically cut down the amount of ultraviolet radiation, but more importantly in the elderly is their habit of not exposing themselves to sunlight, and even if they do many old people will wear broad-brimmed hats to keep the light from their eyes if they have cataracts.

Both dietary and skin sources of vitamin D are important and the elderly frequently suffer a deficiency of each. Vitamin D metabolism may be upset in other ways. In chronic liver disease there will be impairment of hydroxylation of vitamin D_3 to 25-hydroxycholecalciferol. In chronic renal failure there may be failure of 1-hydroxylation of 25-hydroxycholecalciferol to 1,25-dihydroxycholecalciferol (1,25-OH_2-D_3). 1,25-OH_2-D_3 is believed to be the active metabolite and regulates calcium absorption from the gut and the reabsorption of calcium from the renal tubules. Anticonvulsant drugs also interfere with vitamin D metabolism and may cause osteomalacia (Figure 11.2).

Marginal notes: Dietary / Action of ultraviolet light

Clinical features of osteomalacia

The main features of osteomalacia are bone pain and muscular weakness. The bone pains may be generalized and persistent. The pain is probably due to strain on tender soft bone. The muscular weakness is striking and may take the form of a proximal myopathy. There may be difficulty in climbing stairs and the gait is 'waddling'. The shoulder girdle is also affected and there may be difficulty in combing the hair.

The skeleton may be deformed and there is often a kyphosis. Fractures are common, especially of the femoral neck, ribs and scapulae.

Diagnosis of osteomalacia

Marginal note: Radiology

The radiological signs of osteomalacia are characteristic. Pseudo-fractures (Looser's zones) occur most commonly in the scapulae and ribs, but may be in any part of the skeleton; these consist of bands of decalcification obliquely or at right angles to the bone surfaces (Figure 11.3). Other changes are reminiscent of osteoporosis and consist of biconcave vertebral bodies and sometimes crush fractures. The pelvis and the long bones may be deformed and more radio-opaque than normal.

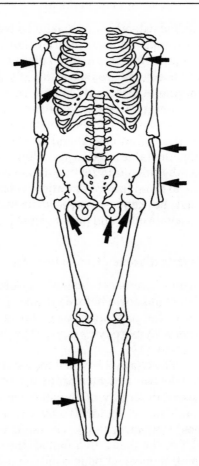

Figure 11.3 Osteomalacia. Sites of Looser's zones

Biochemistry The biochemical changes are variable but characteristic. The plasma calcium level may be normal or low; the serum inorganic phosphorous is usually low and the alkaline phosphatase raised (see Table 11.1). The urinary calcium excretion is low. It is now possible to measure the 25-hydroxycholecalciferol level in the serum by radioimmunoassay in some centres and the finding of a low level is diagnostic of osteomalacia.

Histology   Bone biopsy from the iliac crest may also be diagnostic, but depends on expert histological examination of undecalcified specimens.

Treatment of osteomalacia

Clinical osteomalacia should be treated with calciferol 1.25 mg daily and calcium 1200 mg daily in divided doses initially, whatever the cause of the disease. The symptoms of bone pain and muscular weakness rapidly disappear. The calcium and phosphate levels return to normal in a week or two. The alkaline phosphatase may remain raised for some time, often several months. After a month it should be possible to reduce the dose of vitamin D and calcium, and the BNF vitamin D and calcium tablets (12.5 µg calciferol) once or twice daily are usually adequate for maintenance unless the osteomalacia is due to renal failure or anticonvulsant therapy. A careful watch must be kept for hypercalcaemia. One would expect the Looser's zones and pathological fractures to heal quite rapidly.

Paget's disease of bone (osteitis deformans)

Paget's disease of bone is a disorder of older age groups. It is almost unknown before the age of 40 years, but occurs in about 3% of the population over the age of 60 years. The incidence rises with increasing age and by the ninth decade the incidence is about 11%.

The characteristic features are excessive bone resorption and deposition which occur in a chaotic fashion. This results in severe deformity of the skeleton and the bones are enlarged and highly vascular. It may affect any part of the skeleton, but most frequently the pelvis, tibiae and skull. Sometimes only one half of the pelvis is affected, the other being normal, and in a small number of people only one bone is involved.

The cause of Paget's disease is unknown, but there is a familial tendency which accounts for wide variations of incidence in different communities.

Clinical features of Paget's disease

Asymptomatic Many patients, even with widespread disease, have no symptoms and the diagnosis is only made on X-ray examination for
Pain something else. Generally pain either in the bone, or as a secondary complication of nerve compression, is the major feature

160

Deformity

Nerve
compression

of the disease. Skeletal deformity, such as bowing of the tibia or head enlargement, may be the presenting feature, either associated with pain or not. Bony deformity may lead to foraminal distortion; this most commonly affects the eighth nerve with resultant deafness.

Although the bones are apparently more dense radiologically, the distorted architecture makes them structurally weak. Thus fractures in affected long bones are common, although healing is normal. There may be incomplete stress fractures, especially in a severely bowed tibia on the convex side, which will progress to complete fracture unless action is taken.

Stress
fractures

Rare complications of Paget's disease include the development of osteogenic sarcoma and high output cardiac failure; the latter only occurs when at least a third of the skeleton is involved.

Table 11.1 Biochemical findings in bone disease

Disease	Calcium	Phosphate	Alkaline phosphatase	Acid phosphatase
Osteomalacia	N or ↓	N or ↑	N or ↑	N
Osteoporosis	N	N	N	N
Carcinoma of the prostate	N	N	↑	↑
Myeloma	N	N	N	N
Paget's	N	N	↑	N
Other 2° carcinoma	N	N	↑	N

Diagnostic findings in Paget's disease

Thickening
Rarefaction
Sclerosis

The radiological features of this disease confirm the deformity and enlargement of the affected bones. There is cortical thickening, destruction of the normal trabecular pattern and patches of rarefaction and sclerosis. The disease always starts at one end of the bone and spreads along it. Incomplete fissure fractures may be seen most commonly in the tibia but sometimes in the upper femoral shaft.

Raised
alkaline
phosphatase

Biochemically the alkaline phosphatase is always raised, often very markedly, so if there is a lot of bony involvement. The serum calcium and inorganic phosphate are normal (see Table 11.1). The hydroxyproline levels in the urine are also raised and are a measure of increased bone turnover.

Management of Paget's disease

The great majority of patients with this disease require no

161

treatment since they are asymptomatic. The indications for treatment are fractures, severe bony deformity, and nerve root compression such as deafness and pain. High output cardiac failure rarely occurs without these symptoms, but is an indication for treatment. If patients with Paget's disease are immobilized for any reason there will be increased resorption of bone and consequent hypercalcaemia which will also require treatment even if the patient is otherwise asymptomatic.

Bony pain in Paget's disease can often be controlled with simple analgesics. Root pain and all the other major symptoms of the disease should be treated with calcitonin, which may be extracted from animal or human parathyroid tissue. Porcine or salmon calcitonin (Calcitare, Calsynar) should be given by injection at least five days a week initially in doses between 50 and 100 MRC units daily depending on the severity of the disease. Treatment should be continued in this dosage until the symptoms are relieved and there is a substantial reduction in the serum alkaline phosphatase and urinary hydroxyproline levels. The dose can then be reduced and given at less frequent intervals and often the drug can be stopped for a time and then restarted when symptoms recur. Occasionally there may be sensitivity to these preparations and human calcitonin can be used. There is some evidence that the diphosphonates may be helpful and can improve the control if given with calcitonin.

Malignant deposits in bone

Breast, prostate etc.
There is sometimes difficulty in distinguishing secondary malignant deposits from osteoporosis and Paget's disease. Secondary malignant deposits in bone usually arise from carcinomas of the breast, lung, kidney, thyroid and prostate. These deposits are usually osteolytic, except in the case of prostatic secondaries, which are most often sclerotic. Secondary deposits virtually never occur in the peripheral bones and are most often seen in the spine. The cortex of the bone is often involved, as opposed to osteoporosis where it is not, and there may be erosion of the pedicles. Frequently there is vertebral collapse. Deposits of myeloma in the bones are usually more circumscribed than those of other secondaries and give rise to a 'pepper pot' appearance. In most cases of myeloma the alkaline phosphatase is within normal limits, but in other secondary bony lesions the alkaline phosphatase is raised, which is another feature distinguishing malignant deposits from osteoporosis. Secondary deposits from a carcinoma of the

Myeloma

Carcinoma of prostate

prostate are not uncommon in old men. They are usually sclerotic and sometimes can be mistaken for Paget's disease, but in
Sclerotic the latter there is bony overgrowth and distortion. The acid
deposits phosphatase is usually raised in prostatic carcinomatosis but
not in Paget's. Even widespread deposits from prostatic
carcinoma in bone may cause little in the way of symptoms, but
if they do the commonest problem is pain in the back. Less often
there are symptoms and signs of root compression. The diagnosis is rarely in doubt because of the distinctive appearance of
Needle biopsy the bony secondaries, but if it is, then a needle biopsy of the
prostate will be confirmatory. It is important to establish the
diagnosis of prostatic carcinoma since palliative treatment is
of great benefit. It is now known that very small doses of stilboestrol (1.0 mg three times a day) are effective in shrinking the
deposits, relieving pain and reducing the acid phosphatase
levels. In these small doses stilboestrol causes few side effects
and fluid retention is rarely a problem. Obviously if the prostatic carcinoma is causing symptoms of urinary obstruction
then it will be necessary to remove it surgically by transurethral resection. If the patient is asymptomatic from his secondary
deposits there is no indication for stilboestrol treatment.

The management of other diseases producing secondary
deposits in bone is more difficult. Localized deposits that cause
Other symptoms can be treated by radiotherapy, or, in the case of
secondary nerve root involvement, by nerve block. Many hospitals now
deposits have pain clinics which specialize in this treatment and can
provide very useful relief for the patient. The management of
generalized bony deposits is often less satisfactory, but cytotoxic agents may have a beneficial effect in some cases of
myeloma, and hormone treatment with oestrogens may cause a
worthwhile remission in disseminated breast carcinoma. This
is a specialized area of medicine in which there is promise of
major advances in the future, and it is best to refer the patient
to an oncologist.

Fractures

Fractures of major bones are a common problem in the elderly,
Bone disease because of the increasing incidence of bone disease with age.
The problem is compounded by the increased occurrence of
falls in the elderly (see Chapter 6) and rehabilitation after
fractures is made more difficult by the high level of immobility
and frailty of these patients. Modern attitudes to rehabilitation, together with newer techniques of investigation of

Rehabilitation

bone disease, have brought about a great improvement in the management of fractures. Unfortunately, these advances have not yet become universal but when they do a great deal of suffering, not to mention medical and nursing cost, will be alleviated. The general principle of management of all fractures should be that all patients should be at least as independent after rehabilitation as they were before the injury.

Femur, spine, shoulder

The most important fractures in the elderly are those of the femoral neck, the wrist and the spine; and fracture/dislocation of the humeral neck. In many patients they are associated with the diseases of bone mentioned above and there is a high incidence of other problems, such as cardiovascular and cerebrovascular disease and anaemias. It is essential to identify and treat these problems if the patient is to be successfully rehabilitated. Many fractures in the elderly will be sustained with minimal trauma and even turning over in bed may precipitate a pathological fracture. Thus there is sometimes a delay in diagnosing even major fractures, unless the family physician maintains a high index of suspicion in patients who have 'gone off their feet' or who have taken to their beds.

Femoral neck fractures

Mortality

These are the most serious fractures occurring in the elderly and are very common. The incidence of these fractures rises with increasing age and probably doubles for each 5 year increment after the age of 60 years. By the age of 90 years almost 3% of the population will fracture their femoral neck annually. In people over 65 years the mortality is significant and rises to 60% in those over 95 years. The morbidity in these patients is also very high and on average the length of stay in hospital is about five weeks. Thus the human suffering and the cost implications on health care from this single fracture are enormous. There is no better example of how a modern approach to such a problem can produce enormous benefit.

Prevention

There are several ways in which femoral neck fractures can be prevented. In many instances the causes of falls can be eradicated (see Chapter 6), whether this be by better arrangement of furnishings and fittings in the home or by correction of abnormalities of gait or postural hypotension. Immobility itself is probably a major cause of decalcification in the skeleton and semi-immobile patients are not only more likely to fracture their femurs but are much more difficult to rehabilitate after they have done so and thus the preservation of adequate mobil-

Diagnosis

ity should substantially mitigate the problem of femoral fractures. Prevention can also be helped by prompt identification of any type of bone disease and the family physician is in an ideal position to do this for his elderly patients.

The prompt diagnosis of femoral fractures is not always achieved since the classical features of a history of trauma and pain, together with the signs of shortening and external rotation of the affected leg, are not always obvious. If the fracture is impacted, pain may not be a prime complaint and the patient may just become immobile and stay in bed. Sometimes the inability to stand on the fractured leg may suggest a stroke to the unwary. However, a high index of suspicion and careful examination should always lead to a rapid and accurate diagnosis.

Treatment

Anaemia

The treatment of femoral fractures is always surgical and the patient should immediately be transferred to hospital for X-ray and operative treatment. Internal fixation of the fracture, whether by nail plate or prosthesis, should enable the patient to weight-bear shortly after operation and physiotherapy is the mainstay of rehabilitation. It is also essential to correct the other medical problems that so frequently co-exist in patients with this fracture. Anaemia is the most common problem, whether due to pre-existing anaemia, blood loss into the tissues of two to three pints which may occur at the time of fracture, or to operative blood loss that is inadequately replaced. Many of these patients will have some degree of heart failure or chest infection and these require treatment. Pre-existing neurological problems, such as stroke or Parkinsonism, present special difficulties; but with proper treatment there is no reason why patients should not rapidly regain their previous level of independence. Discharge from hospital should always be aimed for at between two and three weeks after operation and there is no reason why the rehabilitation process should not continue at home, with visits to the physiotherapy department and day hospital as required. From the family physician's point of view it is important to see that adequate rehabilitation is achieved and to ensure that any relevant bone disease is properly treated and followed-up. In the early phase after discharge from hospital it may be necessary to institute extra assistance and support in the home.

Other fractures

Shoulder and
wrist
fractures

The same principles of rehabilitation apply to all fractures, but the ones that are of special interest to the family physician are those of the upper limb; fracture/dislocation of the shoulder and the Colles fracture of the wrist. Although these are often fairly minor disabilities for younger people, in the elderly they may cause major problems, in particular for those living alone. These fractures are not commonly associated with pathological bone disease and although the patients are generally fit, they may be suffering from recurrent falls which require investigation. The majority of these patients can be kept at home, but if there is already some disability or if the patient lives alone it may be advisable to admit them for a short period to a rehabilitation unit or to refer them to the local day hospital.

Summary

Bone disease is very common in the elderly. There is progressive bone loss with age and osteoporosis is extremely prevalent. This is usually generalized and gives rise to backache and predisposes to fractures. Treatment is not completely satisfactory, although calcium and in some cases oestrogens and vitamin D, may be useful. Osteomalacia is less common and extremely difficult to diagnose. However, treatment with vitamin D and calcium is very effective. Paget's disease occurs with increasing frequency with advancing age, but in many cases gives rise to no problems although it may be widespread and severe. Treatment of symptomatic patients with calcitonin can be very beneficial. Malignant deposits in bone occur in many diseases, especially cancers of the breast, lung, prostate, thyroid and kidney. As with other forms of bone disease pathological fractures may occur with minimal trauma; palliative treatment with oestrogens and cytotoxic agents can be of great help in some patients. Fractures are both common and a major source of disability in the elderly. Newer approaches to diagnosis, investigation and rehabilitation have led to a significant reduction in both mortality and especially morbidity in these patients. An active programme of treatment must be instituted at the earliest opportunity, remembering that it should be possible to at least restore the patient to the same level of independence as that obtained before the injury.

12 Disorders of the blood

Hypochromic, microcytic anaemia – Macrocytic and megalo-blastic anaemias – Normocytic, normochromic anaemias – The myeloproliferative syndrome – The gammopathies

Anaemias and other blood disorders are very frequently found in the elderly and, for the most part, are easily recognized, investigated and treated by the family physician. Thus it is important for him to have a firm grasp of the mechanism and investigation of anaemias.

Frequency About 10% of men and 15% of women over 65 years will suffer from anaemia, when this is defined as a haemoglobin value of less than 12.0 g/100 ml. It is frequently considered that haemoglobin levels below this are a normal accompaniment of ageing; but this is not so. There are virtually no specific ageing changes in the blood system and the only major finding is a normal acceleration of the ESR with increasing age. This may be because of the progressive fall of the albumin and relative rise of the globulin values in old age. Since the elderly are able to tolerate anaemia less well than younger patients it is essential to recognize low levels of haemoglobin and to investigate and treat them promptly.

There are few major differences in blood disorders between the elderly and younger people, except in the increased frequency of iron-deficient and megaloblastic anaemias with age and the much more common occurrence of myeloma. Thus this chapter will not involve discussion of haemolytic anaemias and disorders of haemostasis and only brief mention will be made of those leukaemias relevant to the elderly.

167

Symptoms   The symptoms of anaemia in the elderly are generally more marked than in the young. Lethargy, weakness, tiredness and dizziness are common, even in mild anaemia. With more severe degrees of anaemia, falls and symptoms of heart failure occur. Confusion is common especially in megaloblastic anaemias. Apart from palor there is angular stomatitis in deficiency states and atrophic glossitis, especially in pernicious anaemia. Sometimes oedema and other signs of heart failure occur and a systolic murmur may be heard in the aortic area, even in the presence of a normal valve.

Hypochromic, microcytic anaemia

Iron deficiency

This is the most frequently found anaemia and accounts for about one half of all cases. Iron deficiency is the usual cause
Dietary iron lack   and may be precipitated by lack of iron in the diet. This is especially common in those old people who are poor and find that they cannot afford iron-rich food, such as meat and fresh vegetables. Patients who have had a partial gastrectomy also find that iron-containing foods are too indigestible and therefore tend to avoid them from choice. Malabsorption of iron is a less common problem, but may occur in those who have had a gastrectomy or extensive small bowel resection.

Gastro-intestinal bleeding   The major cause of iron deficiency is blood loss, usually from the gastrointestinal tract. This is especially important in the elderly where hiatus hernia, diverticulitis, large bowel carcinoma, piles and the taking of anti-rheumatic drugs that cause gastric bleeding are commonplace. Less often gastric and duodenal ulcers may cause chronic blood loss. All these factors need to be excluded before satisfactory treatment is concluded. Much can be eliminated by a thorough physical examination, including digital examination of the rectum and proctoscopy. If no obvious cause is found, a barium meal and then, if necessary, a barium enema examination must be undertaken. It may be wise to do a sigmoidoscopy as well. To check that blood loss has ceased the faeces should be examined for occult blood on several occasions, since further bleeding is the most frequent
Check for continued blood loss   cause of failure of treatment. Other causes of external blood loss are obvious, but it must be remembered that when the neck of the femur is fractured large quantities of blood are lost into the tissues and are not always efficiently reabsorbed.

Investigation of iron deficiency anaemia

The haemoglobin value and the peripheral blood picture are essential. The anaemia is usually moderate with a haemoglobin value of between 7 and 10 g/100 ml. The serum iron level will be low and the total iron binding capacity increased. The iron saturation will be low. These estimations are important in assessing the degree of iron deficiency and monitoring treatment. The peripheral blood smear will show a hypochromic microcytic picture (see Table 12.1). There is no indication to do a sternal marrow puncture unless other co-existent anaemias are suspected.

As mentioned in the previous paragraph full investigation of the cause of the iron deficiency should be undertaken.

Treatment of iron deficiency

The best treatment of iron deficiency, from whatever cause, is to give oral iron supplements, either ferrous sulphate 200 mg three times daily, or by the slow-release iron preparations such as Feospan 1–2 capsules daily. The latter are probably less efficient methods of giving iron, but this fact is offset by improved tolerability and compliance. If iron by mouth is contra-indicated then it may be given either by intramuscular injection, eg. iron sorbitol citrate (Jectofer) 2 ml daily for about ten days until the iron stores are repleted, or by total dose infusion of iron intravenously. Neither of these parenteral methods of giving iron are more efficient or quicker in replacing the iron stores.

Iron replacement

Causes of treatment failure

The most important reason for failure of treatment is the presence of continued undetected bleeding. It is therefore vital to check for the presence of occult blood in the faeces. Another important cause of treatment failure is inadequate iron replacement, either because insufficient iron has been prescribed, or because the patient does not take the tablets properly. This latter fact is not unusual with oral iron supplements since they have a high incidence of side-effects, such as indigestion and diarrhoea or constipation. If this is suspected then it is better to give parenteral iron. A further cause of treatment failure is the co-existence of other anaemias, such as B_{12} and folate deficiency. More rarely there may be associated pyridoxine deficiency or hypothyroidism.

Macrocytic and megaloblastic anaemias

These are the second commonest causes of anaemia in the elderly. The major problems are deficiency of vitamin B_{12} (pernicious anaemia) or folic acid. Both these substances are stored in the liver and are intimately involved in DNA synthesis and are therefore vital to normal haematopoiesis.

Pernicious anaemia

Vitamin B_{12} is available in meat, some seafoods, eggs and milk. It is absorbed in the terminal part of the ileum provided that there are adequate amounts of intrinsic factor, which itself is produced by the parietal cells in the stomach. Because of its wide availability in foods a dietary deficiency of B_{12} is rare, except in vegetarians and food faddists. The usual cause of deficiency is due to either previous gastric resection or disease, or resections of the terminal ileum, for example in blockage of the lymphatic drainage of the small bowel or Crohn's disease.

Malabsorption of B_{12}

The blood picture in pernicious anaemia will show a macrocytosis and the MCV is raised, usually above 95 femtolitres. The same picture is seen in folic acid deficiency. Because these anaemias tend to be slowly progressive, the haemoglobin value may fall to very low levels before the patient presents himself to the doctor. Thus haemoglobin values as low as 6 g/100 ml are not uncommon (see Table 12.1). With severe macrocytic anaemia there may also be a reduction in both the white blood count and the platelets. In this situation it is vital to send off blood for both serum B_{12} and folate estimation before any treatment is given. If there is any doubt about the diagnosis it is wise to obtain a sternal marrow sample, which will show a megaloblastic picture.

Many patients with pernicious anaemia will have an achlorhydria and also antibodies to parietal cells and thyroglobulins.

Treatment of pernicious anaemia

Vitamin B_{12} must be given by injection and a convenient form is hydroxycyanocobalamin (Neocytamen) 1000 µg. Initially the vitamin should be given daily for a week and after this six-weekly. Because the patient is committed to treatment for life it is important to be absolutely sure of the diagnosis. A useful extra tip is to check the reticulocyte response to treatment at both seven and nine days after the first injection. The reticulocyte rise will be marked and is relative to the level of the initial haemoglobin value. The blood count should be checked twice annually thereafter, for life.

Folic acid deficiency

This is also an important cause of anaemia in the elderly. Folic acid is available in many foods, especially fresh green vegetables, kidney and liver. It is absorbed in the jejunum. The chief causes of folic acid deficiency are dietary and for various reasons old people may not ingest adequate amounts of these foods. This is especially true if they have had a previous gastrectomy. Malabsorption in the jejunum is unusual. Some drugs, most notably phenytoin and phenobarbitone and some of the cytotoxic agents, will interfere with folic acid metabolism and cause deficiency. Liver disease may also contribute to folic acid deficiency. Excessive demands for folate may occur in some malignant diseases and chronic inflammatory states as well as the haemolytic anaemias.

Investigations in suspected folic acid deficiency are the same as for pernicious anaemia and indeed, the two may co-exist. The blood investigations are similar except that the serum folate level will be low.

Treatment of folic acid deficiency is with adequate folic acid replacement. The initial dose of folic acid should be 15 mg daily in divided doses for two to three months or until the body stores are replenished. Thereafter it may be necessary to give a maintenance dose of 5 mg daily if there is still evidence of dietary deficiency or if the patient is taking longterm anticonvulsants.

Other causes of macrocytic anaemia

Liver disease and alcoholism may give rise to a macrocytosis as a result of interference with folic acid and vitamin B_{12} metabolism. Scurvy may also present as a macrocytic anaemia due to deficiency of vitamin C and it may less often cause a hypochromic anaemia. Scurvy may certainly be seen in old men who live alone and eat a diet deficient in fresh fruit and vegetables.

Normocytic, normochromic anaemias

These are rarely severe, and the haemoglobin value is usually above 9 g/100 ml. The usual causes are uraemia due to chronic renal failure and rheumatoid arthritis. A mild anaemia may be seen in polymyalgia rheumatica and temporal arteritis and this responds quickly to steroid treatment. Malignant diseases and chronic infections may produce a normochromic, normocytic anaemia. In these cases the serum iron, B_{12} and folate levels are usually normal.

Table 12.1 Investigation of anaemia

Investigation	Iron deficiency	Pernicious anaemia	Folic acid deficiency
Haemoglobin	7–11 g/100 ml	5–10 g/100 ml	5–10 g/100 ml
MCHC	Low	Normal	Normal
MCV	Normal	High	High
Peripheral blood	Hypochromic, microcytic	Macrocytic	Macrocytic
Serum iron	Low	Normal	Normal
Iron binding capacity	Increased	Normal	Normal
Iron saturation	Low	Normal	Normal
Serum B_{12}	Normal	Low	Normal
Serum folate	Normal	Normal	Low
Marrow sample indicated	No	Sometimes	Sometimes
Antibodies to thyroglobulin	Absent	Usually present	Absent

The myeloproliferative syndrome

This syndrome consists of polycythaemia rubra vera, acute and chronic myeloid leukaemia, essential thrombocythaemia and myelofibrosis. They are not that uncommon in the elderly and have many similar features. In addition there is a certain amount of transition between all of them. The fundamental disorder is in the precursors of the red cells, granulocytes, platelets and fibroblasts.

Polycythaemia

Polycythaemia may be secondary to chronic respiratory disease and some tumours, most notably hypernephroma. It is important to recognize the secondary form since this does not usually require treatment and is not part of the myeloproliferative syndrome, as is primary polycythaemia (rubra vera).

Polycythaemia rubra vera Polycythaemia rubra vera is a chronic condition occurring more often in men than in women in later life. There is overproduction of the red cells, resulting in an increase in the red cell mass. There is also an increase in the blood viscosity; this is important since it predisposes to an increased incidence of peripheral arterial obstruction and transient ischaemic attacks. In some patients there is an increased haemorrhagic tendency. These factors may be very significant in the elderly patient. General complaints may include headaches, shortness of breath, tiredness and dyspepsia. The physical signs are the appearance of high colour and the finding of an enlarged spleen in about two thirds of the patients. The latter finding is important since the spleen is not enlarged in secondary polycythaemia.

Diagnosis The diagnosis of polycythaemia rubra vera is made by the finding of a high haemoglobin, above 19 g/100 ml, a raised PCV, above 54%, and a raised white blood count. The platelet count may also be raised. The red cell alkaline phosphatase and serum B_{12} levels are raised. The distinction must be made from secondary polycythaemia, where the white blood and platelet counts are not raised and the red cell alkaline phosphatase and serum B_{12} levels are normal. In the secondary form the arterial PO_2 is reduced and the PCO_2 is raised (see Table 12.2).

Table 12.2 Differences between primary and secondary polycythaemia

Investigation	Polycythaemia rubra vera	Secondary polycythaemia
Haemoglobin above 19 g/100 ml	Yes	Yes
Packed cell volume > 54%	Yes	Yes
White blood cells and platelets increased	Yes	No
Leucocyte alkaline phosphatase raised	Yes	No
Serum B_{12} raised	Yes	No
Arterial PO_2	Normal	Low
Arterial PCO_2	Normal	Raised
Spleen	Enlarged in 2/3 of patients	Not enlarged

Treatment of polycythaemia rubra vera

Once the diagnosis is established the aim of treatment is to reduce the haematocrit to normal by repeated venesection. Once this has been achieved radioactive phosphorus should be given. The effects will not be apparent for six weeks and the dose may need to be repeated. Frequent venesection will be required and the indications for this are based on the haemoglobin and packed cell volume estimations. Repeated venesection will deplete the body of iron and this may need to be given by oral supplements.

Generally secondary polycythaemia requires no treatment, although in some cases of respiratory failure due to an acute infection a venesection of one pint of blood may be life-saving.

Myelofibrosis (Myelosclerosis)

The bone marrow becomes infiltrated with fibroblasts and fails to perform its normal function. Secondary haematopoiesis then occurs in the liver and spleen and sometimes in other organs. Myelofibrosis may occur as a primary state or be secondary to polycythaemia rubra vera.

The clinical picture is one of increasing anaemia and susceptibility to infections. The liver and the spleen are usually massively enlarged. The lymph nodes may also be enlarged. Sometimes the presentation may be acute left hypochondrial pain and fever due to a splenic infarct.

Investigations   Investigations show that there is universal reduction in red cells, white cells and platelets. The sternal marrow puncture may be difficult and shows a marrow filled with fibroblasts and little in the way of active blood production.

Treatment   There is no effective treatment for myelosclerosis. The best that one can do is to give repeated blood transfusions of fresh blood. Ultimately the patient will die of haemorrhage or overwhelming infection.

Essential thrombocythaemia

This is a rare condition that may be seen in older men. The problem here is that there is an overproduction of platelets, but these do not function normally and bleeding episodes are common. The platelet count is high in the peripheral blood and the bone marrow shows an increase in the megakaryocytes. Treatment is with busulphan (Myeleran) for short-term control, followed by injections of radio-active phosphorus.

Disorders of the blood

Chronic myeloid leukaemia (CML)

This is not frequently seen in older patients and is more a disease of the middle-aged. It may, however, result from polycythaemia rubra vera.

The presenting symptoms are increasing anaemia, recurrent infections and sometimes pain due to the enlargement of the spleen which may be massive. The first sign of the disease may be splenic infarction.

Diagnosis   The diagnosis is made on the peripheral blood count, which shows an anaemia and tremendous increase in the white blood count. The bone marrow examination will confirm the diagnosis when masses of granulocyte precursors are found together with normal mature granulocytes. The Philadelphia chromosome is usually present.

Although the diagnosis is easily made, treatment is not very satisfactory and has shown little improvement in the last few years. Treatment is with busulphan (Myeleran). A careful watch must be made of the peripheral blood count in monitoring the dosage. The prognosis is poor and most patients die within two years. Complete bone marrow suppression may occur with treatment or an acute blast crisis may occur which is usually unresponsive to chemotherapy.

Chronic lymphatic leukaemia

This is principally a disease of the aged. It is caused by a tumour of the precursors of the lymphatic series. Often it is a disease which is very benign, but it may occasionally pursue a more active course and rarely will enter a malignant phase.

Patients usually present with increasing anaemia, but sometimes because of glandular enlargement. Often the disease is discovered by chance when a blood count is done for some other reason. The white count is greatly increased with cells of the lymphatic series. There may be some degree of anaemia. Many glands are usually enlarged and the liver and spleen may be palpable, but not grossly enlarged.

Since many cases run a benign course no treatment is necessary unless the white blood count becomes excessively high (above 300 000), or unless there is evidence of a change to the acute phase of the disease. For more active cases treatment should be given and this is with chlorambucil (Leukeran) 0.2 mg/kg bodyweight per day for about 6 weeks or until there is a good blood count response. Sometimes it is necessary to give steroids if there is anaemia or severe reduction in the platelet count. The majority of patients will survive for a normal span of life.

The gammopathies

These may be mono- or polyclonal. The principal disease is multiple myeloma which is a monoclonal gammopathy. The macroglobulinaemia of Waldenstrom is another rare example of a monoclonal gammopathy.

Multiple myeloma

This is a disseminated malignancy of plasma cells and its incidence occurs increasingly with age. It is characterized by bone destruction, bone marrow failure and the production of large quantities of abnormal globulin which may cause problems with hyperviscosity and become deposited in the kidney amongst other organs.

The clinical features are of bone pain, usually in the spine, due to bone destruction. Sometimes there are neurological signs of both upper and lower motor neurone lesions caused by the bone destruction and infiltration of the tumour. Anaemia is a frequent presentation and renal failure may occur as a result of myeloma deposition in the tubules, calcium deposits due to the hypercalcaemia or uric acid deposits and occasionally, by amyloidosis. These patients are also very susceptible to infections because of the immunoglobulin abnormality.

Diagnosis   The diagnosis is made by finding a very accelerated ESR, usually above 120 mm in the first hour. There is a monoclonal globulin spike of the plasma and urinary electrophoresis and on bone marrow biopsy masses of plasma cells may be seen. The X-ray findings are also characteristic and show well-defined lytic (punched-out) areas in the bones, especially in the spine and skull. The serum immunoglobulins are also abnormal and there is usually a great increase in either IgA, IgG, or IgM.

The natural history of this disease may be very variable. Some patients have no symptoms and may survive for many years without treatment. The majority of cases will be symptomatic and require some treatment. Although there is great variation in life-expectancy the old axiom that there were 'two years without symptoms, two years with symptoms and then death', is probably still true for the majority of elderly patients.

Treatment of myeloma

The first aim of management of this condition is generally supportive. This will include the symptomatic relief of pain by analgesia and by DXT if it is severe and localized. Anaemia should be treated by blood transfusion. Infections should be recognized and treated early. The hypercalcaemia that so often occurs in these patients (in the presence of a normal alkaline phosphatase) should be managed by a high fluid intake, exercises to maintain mobility and by calcitonin injections. Hyperuricaemia can be effectively managed by giving allopurinol (Zyloric) 100 mg three times daily.

Supportive treatment is of little use unless the myeloma is attacked chemically. Although there is some difficulty in exposing elderly patients to longterm, potentially unpleasant treatment, there is now good evidence that intermittent melphalan (Alkeran) 10 mg/m²/day for four days together with prednisolone 60 mg/day once a month will result in some haematological, biochemical and symptomatic improvement in about 60% of cases. The side-effects of this treatment are not too bad and this would be the recommendation for symptomatic elderly patients.

13 Endocrine diseases

The thyroid – Diabetes mellitus – The endocrine disturbances
associated with cancer

The thyroid

Incidence Diseases of the thyroid gland are common in the elderly and
occur in about 3% of those aged over 65 years. Underactivity
of the gland is almost six times more common than overactivity
and men and women are equally affected. This is an area in
geriatric medicine where routine thyroid screening tests have
a great deal of value since unless they are done many cases of
disease will be missed. Symptoms and signs of thyroid disease
may be very vague and the more obvious symptoms that occur
in younger patients may be absent in the elderly. If there is any
question of the diagnosis, a serum T_4 and TSH should be
estimated.

 The thyroid gland synthesizes two major hormones (T_4 and
T_3) from iodine and these are almost entirely protein-bound.
Thus changes in the serum protein levels, common in the old,
will affect the hormonal levels. Although secreted in much
lower concentration, T_3 is probably just as active metabolically
as T_4, from which it is derived by peripheral de-iodination. The
thyroid hormones influence the metabolic activity of all tissues
by increasing the oxygen consumption and heat production.
They also have complex actions on growth, cardiac function
and the metabolism of sugar, fats and proteins. The function of
the thyroid gland is regulated by a negative feed-back system
via the hypothalamus, where thyrotrophin releasing hormone
(TRH) is produced and the anterior part of the pituitary, where

179

thyroid stimulating hormone (TSH) is released. When levels of T_4 and T_3 fall in the serum, increased quantities of TRH and TSH are produced and vice versa.

Tests of thyroid function

In the last few years there has been a change away from the older methods of assessing the protein-bound iodine levels and doing radio-active iodine studies. These tests have been replaced by the more accurate radioimmunoassays of serum T_4 and T_3 which are protein-bound. It is not possible to measure the free or unbound T_4, and to get over this problem the free thyroxine index (FTI) can be calculated by multiplying the serum T_4 by the level of T_3 resin uptake. This, to a large extent, will compensate for the effect of drugs and other factors on the protein-binding. It is also possible to measure the TSH level, and this is fundamental in hypothyroid states, where it is raised. In difficult cases of hyperthyroidism it is possible to measure the TSH response to intravenous TRH injection where there is little or no response of TSH, as opposed to hypothyroidism where the response is exaggerated and prolonged. Finally, it is possible to measure the presence of thyroid antibodies to thyroglobulin, microsomal and nuclear intracellular components. These are important when auto-immune thyroiditis is suspected, such as Hashimoto's disease.

Hypothyroidism (myxoedema)

This is the most important thyroid disorder in the elderly. It is caused by auto-immune thyroiditis (Hashimoto's disease), pituitary insufficiency and also occurs after previous treatment of thyrotoxicosis by radio-active iodine, surgery or anti-thyroid drugs, such as carbimazole. It may present in a variety of ways and a high index of suspicion should be maintained by the family physician, especially since he is at a disadvantage at seeing his patients more regularly than other observers and thus may not notice the changes in appearance that are so typical of myxoedema.

Clinical features   Lethargy, with mental and physical slowness, are cardinal features of hypothyroidism, but these may be mimicked by many other disorders. Sometimes there are major mental changes in hypothyroidism – the so-called 'myxoedema madness'. Constipation is a regular feature. Weight gain is usual, but never marked. Some patients will lose weight because of the markedly decreased appetite. Memory is usually impaired. Intolerance to cold is an important symptom and these patients will wear an inappropriate amount of clothes and often suffer erythema ab igne. Hypothermia is an unusual presentation of hypothyroidism, as is coma. Sometimes the presenting feature may be the carpal tunnel syndrome, where the median nerve to the hand becomes trapped in the oedematous flexor retinaculum of the wrist.

The appearance of a patient with hypothyroidism is characteristic: the face is puffy due to mucoid substances deposited in the skin and there are also mucoid deposits in many other tissues, especially the vocal cords, producing huskiness of the voice and the heart, producing cardiac failure. All the skin is coarse and dry and the hair is similarly affected. The tendon reflexes have a characteristically slow relaxation phase.

Diagnosis The diagnosis is confirmed by finding reduced levels of T_4, T_3 resin uptake and FTI. The TSH level will be high and the auto-antibodies may be raised. The e.c.g. may show many features, such as sinus bradycardia, low voltage complexes, and T wave inversion in advanced cases. The latter is extremely important to recognize since it implies considerable cardiac involvement and should influence treatment.

Treatment of hypothyroidism

The treatment of myxoedema is with replacement thyroxine whatever the cause. Initially one should start with thyroxine 0.05 mg daily. Unless there are any major contraindications, such as obstructive airways disease, it is a good practice to give β-blocker therapy with the thyroxine. Propranolol 10 mg three times daily is usually satisfactory and is mandatory if there are any signs suggestive of myocardial involvement. After two to three weeks the dose of thyroxine should be increased to 0.1 mg daily. After this the increase in thyroxine dosage should be monitored by assessing the serum TSH level. There is no point in doing T_4 estimations in patients who are taking thyroxine. Generally the final replacement dose of thyroxine in the elderly is between 0.1 and 0.15 mg daily. The hormone need only be given once a day. There is no advantage in spreading out the dose and it will only cause failure of drug compliance.

Hyperthyroidism

Clinical features
Overactivity of the thyroid gland usually occurs as a result of uni- or multi-nodular goitres in the elderly. Grave's disease is less common in the older age group than it is in the young. As a result of this the symptoms of thyrotoxicosis may be difficult to evaluate in older patients. There is almost always weight loss, but tremor and agitation are much less frequently seen. Heat intolerance is usually seen in this age group. The eye signs of Grave's disease do not usually occur; thus there will be no proptosis or exophthalmos and lid lag is rarely seen. Atrial fibrillation is a cardinal feature of hyperthyroidism in the elderly. It may not always be established but is quite frequently intermittent, giving rise to palpitations and a rapid ventricular rate. Occasionally hyperthyroidism may be 'masked', when the only findings are weight loss and atrial fibrillation. 'Apathetic' hyperthyroidism also occurs, and in this situation the patients are apathetic rather than agitated and restless, there is weight loss and atrial fibrillation.

Diagnosis
The diagnosis of hyperthyroidism rests upon the clinical picture and the finding of raised thyroid function tests. If there is doubt it may be worth doing a TRH stimulation test, where it will be found that the TSH response to intravenous TRH is little altered or not at all.

Treatment

In the elderly the treatment of choice is with radioactive iodine by mouth. There is rarely any place for carbimazole or surgical treatment as in younger patients. Initially the control of the symptoms of hyperthyroidism are best controlled with β-blocking drugs, and propranolol (Inderal) 10 mg three times daily is usually adequate. If necessary the dose can be increased until the major symptoms of the disease have been controlled. It must be remembered that radioactive iodine treatment takes up to six weeks to be fully effective and β-blockade should be continued for at least that time. The main problem with radioactive iodine is that there is a high incidence of secondary myxoedema, but this can be controlled easily by replacement thyroxine. Patients who have had this form of treatment should be followed-up for life, since the incidence of secondary myxoedema continues to appear for many years after the treatment is given. The TSH level is useful in monitoring this situation.

Non-toxic thyroid goitre

Thyroid goitres may be seen in both hypo- and hyperthyroidism, but many goitres are associated with no abnormality of thyroid function. Sometimes these goitres may be huge. The main cause of non-toxic goitre is iodine-lack in the diet and this occurs sporadically throughout the world. The gland is usually diffusely enlarged. Other causes of non-toxic goitre are auto-immune thyroiditis (Hashimoto's disease) and it is known that some drugs may cause it as well, particularly iodine-containing compounds such as some expectorant mixtures, para-amino salicylic acid and phenylbutazone. The anti-diabetic agent tolbutamide may also cause thyroid enlargement. Any of the anti-thyroid drugs, such as carbimazole and thiouracil will cause thyroid enlargement. The mechanism of goitre production is through an increased output of TSH consequent upon the poor secretion of thyroid hormones.

Carcinomas of the thyroid

These are uncommon conditions in the elderly. The majority are due to papillary carcinoma, but a smaller percentage are due to follicular carcinoma. The natural history of these tumours is extremely variable. They may only be found as an incidental autopsy finding, or they may be extremely malignant, with all degrees of activity between. Local spread is to the lymph nodes in the neck and there may be distant metastases to bone resulting in pathological fractures. They may also metastasize to the lungs and brain. Thyroid cancer should always be suspected in a patient with a single nodule and this is an indication for a radioactive thyroid scan.

The treatment of thyroid cancer is with total thyroidectomy and radioactive iodine. Thyroid replacement hormones should also be given, as some of these tumours are hormone-dependent and it is important to supress TSH production.

Diabetes mellitus

This occurs in at least 2% of the elderly population. There are some features of the disease that do differ from that in younger patients. Ageing changes in the kidney cause a fall in the glomerular filtration rate and a rise in the renal threshold for glucose. Thus many patients who have significant hyperglycaemia will not have glycosuria. It is always essential to perform tests of fasting and post-prandial serum glucose in anyone who is suspected of having diabetes. Fasting blood sugars above 7.0 mmol/l and any random blood sugar level above 10.5 mmol/l indicates that the patient has diabetes.

Long-standing diabetes
Many patients will have survived into old age with long-standing diabetes, and most of these will be insulin-dependent. Apart from the usual complications of long-standing diabetes, such as peripheral neuropathy and the eye changes of cataract and retinopathy, there are no particular problems in these patients.

Late onset diabetes
Similarly many old patients will have the classical symptoms of diabetes for the first time: excessive thirst, polyuria and weight loss, sometimes with infections, particularly of the urinary tracts and pruritis. This is typical of late onset diabetes and the patients respond well to treatment with carbohydrate restricted diet and, if necessary, anti-diabetic drugs. Rarely will they require insulin, except in the situation where there is a serious intercurrent infection or where operation is necessary.

Treatment

The drug of first choice is tolbutamide (Rastinon) 1.0–2.0 g daily in divided doses if the patient does not respond adequately to a restricted carbohydrate diet. Not too much note should be taken of the urine sugars, since there is often a high renal threshold for sugar. Blood sugars should always be monitored regularly. If tolbutamide fails to control the disease glibenclamide (Daonil) 5–15 mg daily or chlorpropamide (Diabenese) 100–350 mg daily should be used in a once a day dose. In obese mild diabetic patients there may be a place for metformin (Glucophage) 500–1700 mg daily either on its own or in combination with another anti-diabetic drug. The use of phenformin (Dibotin) is not recommended now because of its propensity to cause lactic acidosis. Confusional states and other mental changes may occur commonly in diabetics and may be a result of either hyperglycaemia or, more commonly, hypoglycaemia.

A significant proportion of diabetics will present for the first time in later life with major infections, gangrene of the legs, peripheral neuritis or even coma. The family physician must always be aware of this possibility and the use of blood glucose testing papers (Dextrostix) should be in every medical bag.

184

Iatrogenic
factors

It is important to remember that all the diuretic agents may cause some glucose intolerance and may light up existing diabetes or precipitate a new case. The corticosteroid drugs will have the same effect to an even greater extent. There is also evidence that glucose metabolism may be upset after myocardial infarction and glycosuria also occurs frequently after subarachnoid haemorrhage.

Hyperosmolar
pre-coma

Hyperosmolar non-ketoacidotic diabetic pre-coma or coma is an unusual but serious condition in the elderly. In this situation the blood sugar rises to very high levels without many of the warning signs of diabetic coma. Indeed, coma occurs at a very late stage in the illness. These patients are profoundly acidotic and dehydrated and are generally very sensitive to small doses of insulin. They require immediate transfer to hospital, where the mainstay of treatment is to correct the acidosis and the dehydration with hypotonic saline.

Complications

With proper understanding of the disease patients with diabetes should present no major problems for the family physician. The eye complications of cataract and retinopathy require referral to an ophthalmologist. It is also important to remember that uncontrolled sugar levels will alter the refraction of the eye and these patients may well complain of misty vision. Pressure sores and diabetic ulcers require careful treatment of the local condition as well as of the diabetic state. Any signs of incipient gangrene of the feet should indicate immediate referral to a vascular surgeon. Attention should be paid to foot care in these patients and a chiropodist should be involved. Finally, if there are any difficulties in blood sugar control at home it is probably better to admit the patient to hospital, where it may be useful to put the patient on twice daily soluble insulin in order to establish proper control before going back to oral hypoglycaemic agents.

The endocrine disturbances associated with cancer

Abnormal hormone secretions associated with some cancers used to be thought of as rare. We now know that this is not the case, and some cancers, in particular oat cell carcinoma of the bronchus, are frequently associated with ectopic and inappropiate hormone production.

ACTH production

One half of all oat cell carcinomas of the bronchus will result in abnormal ACTH production. The same situation may be caused by phaeochromocytomas and islet cell tumours of the pancreas. The clinical syndrome produced is like Cushing's disease. There is muscular weakness and glucose intolerance, often amounting to diabetes mellitus. The serum sodium levels are high and the potassium low. There is also an alkalosis.

The treatment is ideally to remove the primary tumour, either by surgical resection or by deep X-ray therapy. It may be necessary to perform a medical adrenalectomy or to give chemotherapy. The biochemical results of these procedures are usually satisfactory.

Antidiuretic hormone (ADH) secretion

About 40% of oat cell bronchial carcinomas will lead to inappropriate ADH secretion. In this situation there is an inappropriate anti-diuresis and this results in a dilutional hyponatraemia with drowsiness and confusion. Most of these patients respond well to water restriction, but, if possible, the primary tumour should be removed.

Parathyroid hormone (PTH) secretion

Any squamous cell carcinoma or adenocarcinoma of the kidney may produce excessive amounts of PTH. This may occur without any evidence of bony metastases. The result is significant hypercalcaemia. This in turn leads to vomiting, polydipsia and polyuria. Psychotic changes may also occur. If possible the primary tumour should be removed. The hypercalcaemia is best treated with calcitonin 100 units daily by injection. Sometimes oral aspirin and indomethazine may be effective.

Summary

Thyroid disease is an important condition in older people. Hypothyroidism is common and may easily be missed if a high index of suspicion is not maintained. The serum T_4 and TSH levels should be estimated in any patient complaining of physical and mental slowness, especially if there is also a bradycardia and slowing of the relaxation phase of the tendon jerks. Hypothyroidism may be 'masked' or 'apathetic' in the elderly and the usual signs of excessive agitation, tremor and proptosis normally seen in younger patients may be absent. Virtually all these elderly patients have atrial fibrillation, which is usually rapid and often intermittent. Treatment in the first instance is with β-blocking agents in sufficient dosage to control the symptoms and then with radioactive iodine. As many as a third of these patients ultimately develop hypothyroidism and therefore should be followed-up indefinitely.

Diabetes mellitus is a common disease in the elderly and may be caused by both diuretic agents and corticosteroids. Control is often satisfactory with diet and weight control alone, but many patients require oral hypoglycaemic agents as well. If there are any problems with control, twice daily soluble insulin may be helpful. Special attention must be paid to foot care, control of infections and the possibility of gangrene, eye problems and peripheral neuritis.

The more esoteric endocrine problems of some cancers, especially oat cell carcinoma of the bronchus are discussed and should be recognized by the family physician.

Index